REVERSE TYPE 2 DIABETES IN 30 DAYS

Guidelines For You To Prevent, Control, Maintain and Eradicate Type 2 Diabetes Completely Through Simple Dieting and Lifestyles(Dos and Don'ts, Risk factors to avoid, Handling Stigmatization)

By

LAURA D. VANDERGRIFF

CONTENTS

Introduction

- ➢ Key nutrients and their effects on blood sugar levels
- ➢ Physical activity and exercise
- ➢ Benefits of regular exercise
- ➢ Types of exercise suitable for individuals with diabetes
- ➢ Incorporating physical activity into daily routine
- ➢ Weight management and its impact on diabetes
- ➢ Strategies for achieving and maintaining a healthy weight
- ➢ Understanding the link between obesity and diabetes

3. Blood Sugar Control
- ➢ Monitoring blood glucose levels
- ➢ Importance of regular monitoring
- ➢ Techniques for accurate measurement
- ➢ Medications and insulin therapy
- ➢ Overview of common diabetes medications
- ➢ Insulin therapy and its role in managing diabetes

- ➢ Alternative therapies and complementary approaches
- ➢ Herbal remedies and supplements
- ➢ Mind-body techniques for stress management and blood sugar control

4. Support and Lifestyle Changes
- ➢ The role of healthcare professionals in diabetes reversal
- ➢ Building a support system
- ➢ Family and friends
- ➢ Diabetes support groups and communities
- ➢ Coping with the emotional aspects of diabetes
- ➢ Dealing with frustration, fear, and stigma
- ➢ Techniques for improving mental well-being

5. Long-Term Maintenance and Prevention
- ➢ Strategies for maintaining diabetes reversal
- ➢ Continuing healthy habits

➤ Regular check-ups and follow-ups
➤ Preventing the onset of type 2 diabetes
➤ Lifestyle changes for high-risk individuals
➤ Early detection and intervention

Conclusion
A. Recap of key points
B. Encouragement and motivation for readers on their journey to reverse type 2 diabetes

Introduction

Type 2 diabetes is a chronic metabolic disorder characterized by high blood sugar levels, impaired insulin function, and insulin resistance. It is a prevalent health condition affecting millions of people worldwide and has emerged as a significant public health concern. Unlike type 1 diabetes, which is typically diagnosed in childhood and results from an autoimmune response, type 2 diabetes primarily develops in adulthood and is strongly associated with lifestyle factors.

The global prevalence of type 2 diabetes has been steadily rising over the past few decades, fueled by sedentary lifestyles, unhealthy dietary choices, and increasing rates of obesity. It is no longer confined to older adults; younger individuals, including adolescents and even children, are increasingly being diagnosed with this condition. This alarming trend highlights the urgent need for understanding and addressing the root causes of type 2 diabetes.

Type 2 diabetes poses serious health risks and complications if left uncontrolled. Elevated blood sugar levels can lead to damage in various organs, including the heart, blood vessels, kidneys, eyes, and nerves. Individuals with uncontrolled diabetes are at a higher risk of cardiovascular diseases, stroke, kidney failure, blindness, and lower limb amputations.

However, the good news is that type 2 diabetes is largely preventable and even reversible through lifestyle modifications. By adopting healthy habits and making positive changes in diet, exercise, and overall lifestyle, individuals can regain control over their blood sugar levels, reduce their dependency on medication, and improve their overall health and well-being.

This book aims to provide a comprehensive guide for reversing type 2 diabetes by addressing its underlying causes and equipping individuals with the knowledge and tools necessary to make sustainable lifestyle changes. It will delve into the role of nutrition, exercise, weight management, blood sugar monitoring, medication, and alternative therapies. Additionally, it will explore the importance of emotional support, building a strong support system, and long-term maintenance to ensure continued success.

By empowering readers with evidence-based information, practical strategies, and inspiring success stories, this book aims to guide them on their journey towards reversing type 2 diabetes and achieving a healthier, happier life. It is time to take control of your health and overcome the challenges of type 2 diabetes.

The prevalence and impact of type 2 diabetes

❖ Prevalence:

Global Prevalence: Type 2 diabetes has reached epidemic proportions worldwide. According to the International Diabetes Federation (IDF), as of 2021, approximately 463 million adults (20-79 years) were living with diabetes globally, and around 90% of them had type 2 diabetes.

Increasing Incidence: The prevalence of type 2 diabetes has been rising rapidly in recent years, primarily due to sedentary lifestyles, unhealthy diets, and increasing obesity rates. The aging population and genetic predisposition also contribute to its prevalence.

❖ Impact:

Health Consequences: Type 2 diabetes can lead to various health complications, both acute and chronic. These include cardiovascular diseases (heart attack, stroke), kidney disease, nerve damage (neuropathy), eye problems (retinopathy), foot ulcers, and an increased risk of infections. If left uncontrolled, it can significantly reduce the quality of life and even lead to premature death.

Economic Burden: Type 2 diabetes poses a substantial economic burden on healthcare systems, individuals, and society. The costs include medical expenses, such as hospitalizations, medications, and regular monitoring, as well as indirect costs like reduced productivity, missed workdays, and disability benefits. The IDF estimated that in 2019, the global healthcare expenditure related to diabetes reached $760 billion.

Reduced Life Expectancy: Type 2 diabetes is associated with reduced life expectancy, primarily due to its complications. Poorly managed diabetes can increase the risk of developing other chronic conditions and lead to premature mortality.

Impact on Mental Health: Living with a chronic condition like type 2 diabetes can have psychological implications. The disease requires significant lifestyle changes, strict management, and monitoring, which can lead to stress, anxiety, depression, and reduced overall well-being.

Public Health Challenge: Type 2 diabetes presents a significant public health challenge as it contributes to the increasing burden of non-communicable diseases (NCDs). It requires comprehensive strategies for prevention, early detection, and effective management to reduce its impact on individuals and society.

Addressing the prevalence and impact of type 2 diabetes requires a multi-faceted approach, including promoting healthy lifestyles, improving access to healthcare and education, implementing policies to prevent obesity, and ensuring early diagnosis and appropriate management of the disease.

The importance of addressing the root causes

Addressing the root causes of type 2 diabetes is crucial for several reasons. By targeting the underlying factors that contribute to the development of the disease, we can have a significant impact on its prevalence and reduce the burden on individuals, healthcare systems, and society. Here are the key reasons why addressing the root causes of type 2 diabetes is important:

Prevention: Type 2 diabetes is largely preventable, especially when the root causes are addressed. By focusing on promoting healthy lifestyles, including regular physical activity, balanced diets, and weight management, we can prevent or delay the onset of type 2 diabetes in many individuals. Prevention efforts can help reduce the number of new cases and the associated health and economic burden.

Improved Health Outcomes: Managing type 2 diabetes requires long-term care and monitoring. By addressing the root causes, such as obesity, sedentary behavior, and poor dietary choices, we can improve overall health outcomes for individuals with the disease. This includes better glycemic control, reduced risk of complications, and enhanced quality of life.

Cost Savings: Type 2 diabetes imposes a significant economic burden on healthcare systems and society. By targeting the root causes, we can potentially reduce the need for expensive medical interventions and long-term management. Prevention and lifestyle interventions are often cost-effective strategies that can result in substantial cost savings in the long run.

Promoting Healthy Communities: Addressing the root causes of type 2 diabetes involves creating environments that support and promote healthy behaviors. This includes improving access to nutritious food options, creating safe spaces for physical activity, and implementing policies that encourage healthy choices. By doing so, we can create healthier communities that benefit not only individuals at risk of type 2 diabetes but the entire population.

Holistic Approach to Health: Type 2 diabetes is influenced by a complex interplay of genetic, behavioral, and environmental factors. By addressing the root causes, we adopt a holistic approach to health that recognizes the interconnectedness of various factors. This approach not only benefits individuals with diabetes but also promotes overall health and well-being.

Reducing the Burden of Non-communicable Diseases: Type 2 diabetes is one of the leading contributors to the global burden of non-communicable diseases (NCDs). By addressing its root causes, we tackle not only diabetes but also other related NCDs such as cardiovascular diseases and obesity. This comprehensive approach can have a far-reaching impact on public health and reduce the overall burden of NCDs.

Addressing the root causes of type 2 diabetes requires a multi-sectoral approach involving individuals, communities, healthcare systems, policymakers, and other stakeholders. By focusing on prevention, health promotion, and creating supportive environments, we can make significant strides in combating type 2 diabetes and improving overall health outcomes.

Overview of the book's approach and goals

Overview:

"Managing Type 2 Diabetes" is a comprehensive book that provides a holistic approach to understanding and managing type 2 diabetes. The book aims to empower individuals with knowledge and practical strategies to prevent the onset of type 2 diabetes, effectively manage the condition if already diagnosed, and improve overall health and well-being.

Approach:

Education and Awareness: The book begins by providing a clear and concise overview of type 2 diabetes, including its causes, risk factors, and the physiological mechanisms involved. It emphasizes the importance of understanding the disease to make informed decisions and take proactive steps towards prevention and management.

Prevention Strategies: The book emphasizes the significance of prevention and offers evidence-based strategies to reduce the risk of developing type 2 diabetes. It explores lifestyle modifications, such as healthy eating, regular physical activity, weight management, and stress reduction techniques. It provides practical tips and guidance on implementing these changes effectively.

Medical Management: For individuals already diagnosed with type 2 diabetes, the book delves into the medical management aspects. It provides information on various treatment options, including oral medications, insulin therapy, and other adjunctive therapies. It emphasizes the importance of regular monitoring, self-care practices, and medication adherence for optimal glycemic control.

Lifestyle Modifications: Recognizing the critical role of lifestyle in managing type 2 diabetes, the book explores in-depth the various lifestyle modifications that can have a positive impact on the condition. It provides guidance on developing healthy eating habits, creating an exercise routine, managing stress, improving sleep, and incorporating self-care practices into daily life.

Emotional and Mental Well-being: The book acknowledges the emotional and mental impact of living with type 2 diabetes and offers strategies to cope with the challenges. It addresses topics such as stress management, dealing with diabetes-related emotions, maintaining a positive mindset, and seeking support from healthcare professionals and support networks.

Long-term Complications and Risk Reduction: Understanding the potential complications associated with type 2 diabetes, the book highlights the importance of long-term risk reduction. It provides information on monitoring and managing common complications such as cardiovascular disease, kidney problems, neuropathy, and eye complications. It offers guidance on lifestyle and medical interventions to minimize the risk of these complications.

Goals:

To provide comprehensive information about type 2 diabetes, empowering readers with knowledge and understanding of the disease.

To emphasize the importance of prevention and provide practical strategies to reduce the risk of developing type 2 diabetes.

To guide individuals diagnosed with type 2 diabetes in managing the condition effectively through lifestyle modifications, medication management, and self-care practices.

To address the emotional and mental well-being of individuals with type 2 diabetes and provide tools for coping with the challenges.
To promote long-term risk reduction by educating readers about potential complications and offering guidance on minimizing their occurrence.

Overall, "Managing Type 2 Diabetes" is a comprehensive guide that combines scientific knowledge with practical advice to empower individuals in the prevention, management, and overall well-being while living with type 2 diabetes.

Understanding Type 2 Diabetes

Insulin Resistance: In individuals with type 2 diabetes, the cells in their body become resistant to the action of insulin. This means that even though insulin is present, it becomes less effective in facilitating the entry of glucose into the cells. As a result, glucose remains in the bloodstream, leading to high blood sugar levels.

Insufficient Insulin Production: Over time, the pancreas may also fail to produce enough insulin to overcome the insulin resistance. This further contributes to elevated blood sugar levels.

Risk Factors:
Several risk factors increase the likelihood of developing type 2 diabetes:

Obesity or excess body weight, particularly abdominal or visceral fat.

Sedentary lifestyle and lack of regular physical activity.

Unhealthy eating habits, especially a diet high in refined carbohydrates and sugar.

Family history of diabetes.

Age (risk increases with age, particularly after 45 years).

Ethnicity (certain populations, such as African Americans, Hispanics, and Asians, have a higher risk).

Symptoms:

Type 2 diabetes may initially present without noticeable symptoms, or the symptoms may be mild and develop gradually. Common symptoms include:

Frequent urination
Increased thirst
Unexplained weight loss or gain
Fatigue or weakness
Blurred vision

Slow healing of wounds or infections
Tingling or numbness in the hands or feet (neuropathy)

Diagnosis:
Diagnosis of type 2 diabetes is typically made through blood tests that measure fasting blood sugar levels or levels after consuming a glucose-rich drink. A glycated hemoglobin (HbA1c) test may also be used to assess average blood sugar levels over the past few months.

Management:
Managing type 2 diabetes involves a combination of lifestyle modifications, medication, and regular monitoring. Key aspects include:

Healthy Eating: Adopting a balanced diet rich in whole grains, lean proteins, fruits, vegetables, and healthy fats. Monitoring carbohydrate intake is crucial to managing blood sugar levels.

Regular Physical Activity: Engaging in moderate-intensity aerobic exercises, such as walking, swimming, or cycling, for at least 150 minutes per week. Strength training and flexibility exercises are also beneficial.

Medication: In some cases, medication may be prescribed to help control blood sugar levels. Common medications include oral antidiabetic drugs, insulin injections, or a combination of both.

Blood Sugar Monitoring: Regularly monitoring blood sugar levels using a glucose meter to ensure they are within the target range. This helps in making informed decisions about lifestyle adjustments and medication.

Complications:
Poorly managed type 2 diabetes can lead to various long-term complications, including:

Cardiovascular diseases (heart attacks, strokes)
Kidney disease (nephropathy)
Nerve damage (neuropathy)
Eye problems (retinopathy)
Foot problems, including infections and ulcers

Prevention:
Type 2 diabetes is largely preventable through healthy lifestyle choices, such as maintaining a healthy weight, engaging in regular physical activity, and adopting a balanced diet. Preventive measures also include regular health check-ups, managing stress levels, and avoiding tobacco use.

Understanding type 2 diabetes is crucial for early detection, effective management, and prevention. By adopting a proactive approach to lifestyle choices and seeking appropriate medical care, individuals can live well with type 2 diabetes and reduce the risk of complications.

Definition and causes of type 2 diabetes

Type 2 diabetes is a chronic metabolic disorder characterized by high blood sugar levels (hyperglycemia) resulting from a combination of insulin resistance and insufficient insulin production. It is the most common form of diabetes, accounting for the majority of diabetes cases worldwide.

Causes of Type 2 Diabetes:

Insulin Resistance: Insulin resistance is a key factor in the development of type 2 diabetes. It occurs when the body's cells become less responsive to the action of insulin. As a result, glucose (sugar) is not effectively transported from the bloodstream into the cells, leading to elevated blood sugar levels.

Insufficient Insulin Production: While insulin resistance is a primary cause of type

2 diabetes, there is also often an associated deficiency in insulin production. The pancreas, which produces insulin, may not be able to produce enough insulin to compensate for the insulin resistance. This inadequate insulin production further contributes to elevated blood sugar levels.

Genetic Factors: Type 2 diabetes has a significant genetic component. Certain genetic variations can increase an individual's susceptibility to developing the condition. Having a family history of type 2 diabetes is a known risk factor, indicating the potential influence of genetic factors in its development.

Lifestyle Factors: Unhealthy lifestyle choices play a significant role in the development of type 2 diabetes. These factors include:

Obesity: Excess body weight, particularly abdominal or visceral fat, increases the risk of developing insulin resistance.

Sedentary Lifestyle: Lack of regular physical activity reduces insulin sensitivity and contributes to insulin resistance.

Poor Diet: A diet high in refined carbohydrates, sugary foods, and unhealthy fats can contribute to insulin resistance and weight gain.

Age and Ethnicity: Type 2 diabetes risk increases with age, particularly after 45 years. Certain ethnic groups, such as African Americans, Hispanics, Asians, and Native Americans, have a higher predisposition to developing the condition.

Gestational Diabetes: Women who have had gestational diabetes (diabetes during pregnancy) have an increased risk of developing type 2 diabetes later in life.

It's important to note that while these factors contribute to the development of type 2 diabetes, the exact interplay between genetic and environmental factors is complex and not yet fully understood. Nonetheless, adopting a healthy lifestyle, maintaining a healthy weight, and regular monitoring can help reduce the risk and effectively manage type 2 diabetes.

Risk factors and common misconceptions

Risk Factors of Type 2 Diabetes:

Obesity or Excess Weight: Being overweight or obese significantly increases the risk of developing type 2 diabetes. Excess body fat, particularly abdominal or visceral fat, is closely associated with insulin resistance.

Sedentary Lifestyle: Lack of physical activity and a sedentary lifestyle contribute to insulin resistance and increase the risk of type 2 diabetes. Regular exercise improves insulin sensitivity and helps maintain a healthy weight.

Unhealthy Diet: Consuming a diet high in refined carbohydrates, added sugars, and unhealthy fats can contribute to weight gain, insulin resistance, and the development of type 2 diabetes. A diet rich in whole grains, fruits, vegetables, lean proteins, and healthy fats is recommended for reducing the risk.

Family History and Genetics: Having a close family member, such as a parent or sibling, with type 2 diabetes increases the risk of developing the condition. Genetic factors play a role in determining an individual's susceptibility to type 2 diabetes.

Age: The risk of type 2 diabetes increases with age, particularly after the age of 45. This is partly due to reduced physical activity, muscle loss, and changes in metabolism that occur as people age.

Ethnicity: Certain ethnic groups have a higher risk of developing type 2 diabetes. This includes individuals of African, Hispanic, Asian, and Native American descent.

Gestational Diabetes: Women who have had gestational diabetes (diabetes during pregnancy) have an increased risk of developing type 2 diabetes later in life.

Common Misconceptions of Type 2 Diabetes:

Misconception: Type 2 diabetes only affects older adults.

Reality: While the risk increases with age, type 2 diabetes can develop at any age, including in children and young adults.

Misconception: Type 2 diabetes is caused by eating too much sugar.

Reality: While a diet high in added sugars can contribute to weight gain and increased risk, type 2 diabetes is a complex condition influenced by various factors, including genetics, lifestyle, and obesity.

Misconception: People with type 2 diabetes can't eat any carbohydrates.

Reality: Carbohydrates should be consumed in moderation, but they are an important part of a balanced diet. The focus should be on choosing whole grains, fruits, and vegetables while managing portion sizes and monitoring blood sugar levels.

Misconception: Only overweight or obese people develop type 2 diabetes.

Reality: While excess weight is a significant risk factor, not everyone with type 2 diabetes is overweight. Thin or normal-weight individuals can also develop the condition due to genetic factors and other risk factors.

Misconception: Type 2 diabetes can be cured by simply losing weight.

Reality: While weight loss can improve insulin sensitivity and blood sugar control, type 2 diabetes is a chronic condition that requires long-term management. Sustainable lifestyle changes, medication, and regular monitoring are often necessary.

Misconception: People with type 2 diabetes can't lead a normal life.

Reality: With proper management, people with type 2 diabetes can lead active and fulfilling lives. Lifestyle modifications, medication, and regular check-ups enable individuals to effectively control blood sugar levels and minimize the risk of complications.

It's important to dispel misconceptions about type 2 diabetes and promote accurate understanding to encourage prevention, early detection, and effective management of the condition.

Consequences of uncontrolled diabetes on health

Uncontrolled diabetes can have significant consequences on a person's health, affecting various organs and systems in the body. Here are some of the potential consequences:

Cardiovascular Complications: Uncontrolled diabetes increases the risk of cardiovascular diseases, including heart attacks, strokes, and peripheral arterial disease. Elevated blood sugar levels, combined with other risk factors such as high blood pressure and high cholesterol, can damage blood vessels and contribute to the development of atherosclerosis (narrowing of the arteries).

Kidney Disease (Nephropathy): Prolonged high blood sugar levels can damage the kidneys' filtering units, leading to diabetic nephropathy. This condition impairs kidney function and can progress to chronic kidney disease and end-stage renal disease, requiring dialysis or kidney transplantation.

Eye Complications (Retinopathy): Uncontrolled diabetes can cause damage to the small blood vessels in the retina, leading to diabetic retinopathy. This condition can result in vision loss and blindness if left untreated.

Nerve Damage (Neuropathy): Chronic high blood sugar levels can damage nerves throughout the body, causing diabetic neuropathy. Symptoms may include numbness, tingling, pain, or weakness, typically affecting the feet and legs.

Neuropathy can also affect the digestive system, urinary tract, and other organs.

Foot Problems: Diabetes-related nerve damage and reduced blood circulation can increase the risk of foot problems. Poorly healing foot ulcers and infections can develop, potentially leading to severe complications, such as gangrene and amputation.

Increased Infection Risk: Uncontrolled diabetes can weaken the immune system, making individuals more susceptible to infections. Common infections include skin infections, urinary tract infections, and fungal infections.

Dental Issues: Diabetes can increase the risk of gum disease (periodontitis) and other dental problems. Poorly controlled blood sugar levels can impair the body's ability to fight bacterial infections, leading to oral health complications.

Sexual and Reproductive Issues: Uncontrolled diabetes can contribute to sexual dysfunction in both men and women. In men, it can lead to erectile dysfunction, while women may experience vaginal dryness and reduced libido. Poorly controlled diabetes during pregnancy can also increase the risk of complications for both the mother and the baby.

Mental Health Challenges: Living with uncontrolled diabetes can be emotionally challenging and increase the risk of mental health issues such as depression and anxiety. The burden of managing the condition, potential complications, and lifestyle adjustments can impact a person's well-being.

Increased Risk of Other Conditions: Uncontrolled diabetes is associated with an increased risk of other health problems, including certain types of cancer, sleep apnea, fatty liver disease, and cognitive decline.

It is crucial to manage diabetes effectively through lifestyle modifications, medication, regular monitoring, and regular healthcare check-ups to minimize the risk of complications and maintain overall health and well-being.

2

Lifestyle Modifications for Reversal

Lifestyle modifications play a crucial role in the management and potential reversal of type 2 diabetes. These changes focus on improving insulin sensitivity, promoting weight loss, and maintaining healthy blood sugar levels. Here are some key lifestyle modifications that can help in the reversal of type 2 diabetes:

Healthy Eating

Follow a Balanced Diet: Adopt a balanced diet that includes a variety of whole grains, lean proteins, healthy fats, and plenty of fruits and vegetables.

Portion Control: Be mindful of portion sizes to manage calorie intake and blood sugar levels effectively.

Limit Refined Carbohydrates and Added Sugars: Minimize or avoid processed foods, sugary drinks, sweets, and foods with high glycemic index that can cause blood sugar spikes.

Focus on Fiber: Include high-fiber foods like whole grains, legumes, and vegetables, as they help regulate blood sugar levels and promote satiety.

Regular Physical Activity:

Aim for Aerobic Exercise: Engage in moderate-intensity aerobic activities such as brisk walking, cycling, swimming, or dancing for at least 150 minutes per week.
Include Strength Training: Incorporate strength training exercises at least twice a week to build muscle mass and improve insulin sensitivity.

Stay Active Throughout the Day: Avoid prolonged sitting and aim for regular movement and activity throughout the day. Weight Management:

Lose Excess Weight: Achieve and maintain a healthy weight through a combination of a balanced diet and regular physical activity. Weight loss can significantly improve insulin sensitivity and blood sugar control.

Focus on Abdominal Fat Reduction: Reduce visceral fat (fat around the abdomen) as it is strongly associated with insulin resistance. This can be achieved through a combination of diet, exercise, and overall weight loss.

Stress Management:

Practice Stress-Relieving Techniques: Engage in activities like meditation, deep breathing exercises, yoga, or hobbies to manage stress levels effectively. Chronic stress can affect blood sugar control.

Adequate Sleep:

Prioritize Sleep: Aim for 7-8 hours of quality sleep each night. Poor sleep quality and duration can affect insulin sensitivity and glucose metabolism.
Regular Monitoring and Support:

Monitor Blood Sugar Levels: Regularly monitor blood glucose levels to track progress and make adjustments to lifestyle modifications or treatment plans as needed.

Seek Professional Support: Work with healthcare professionals, such as doctors, dietitians, or diabetes educators, who can provide guidance, education, and ongoing support in managing and potentially reversing type 2 diabetes.

It's important to note that lifestyle modifications should be personalized to individual needs and preferences. Before making any significant changes, it is advisable to consult with a healthcare professional who can provide personalized recommendations based on your specific health condition and requirements.

Importance of diet in managing diabetes

The importance of diet in managing diabetes cannot be overstated. A well-planned and balanced diet plays a crucial role in controlling blood sugar levels, preventing complications, and promoting overall health for individuals with diabetes.

Here are some key reasons why diet is essential in managing diabetes:

Blood sugar control: The primary goal of dietary management in diabetes is to regulate blood glucose levels. By choosing the right foods and controlling portion sizes, individuals can help keep their blood sugar within a healthy range. Foods with a low glycemic index, such as whole grains, vegetables, and legumes, are typically recommended as they cause a gradual and steady rise in blood sugar levels.

Weight management: Maintaining a healthy weight is important for managing diabetes, as excess body weight can increase insulin resistance and lead to higher blood sugar levels. A balanced diet that focuses on portion control, calorie moderation, and nutrient density can help individuals achieve and maintain a healthy weight, reducing the risk of complications associated with diabetes.

Prevention and management of complications: Diabetes can lead to various complications, such as heart disease, stroke, kidney disease, nerve damage, and eye problems. A healthy diet can significantly reduce the risk of these complications. For example, a diet low in saturated and trans fats, cholesterol, and sodium can help prevent heart disease and high blood pressure, which are common in individuals with diabetes.

Energy and nutrient supply: Proper nutrition is essential to provide the body with the energy and nutrients it needs to function optimally. A balanced diet that includes a variety of foods from different food groups ensures an adequate intake of carbohydrates, proteins, healthy fats, vitamins, minerals, and fiber. These nutrients support overall health, enhance immune function, promote wound healing, and reduce the risk of infections, which is particularly important for individuals with diabetes, as they may have impaired healing and a higher susceptibility to infections.

Blood pressure and cholesterol management: People with diabetes are at an increased risk of developing high blood pressure and abnormal cholesterol levels. A healthy diet, rich in fruits, vegetables, whole grains, lean proteins, and healthy fats, can help manage blood pressure and cholesterol levels. Consuming foods high in fiber, such as oats, legumes, and vegetables, can be especially beneficial in controlling cholesterol.

Individualized meal planning: Diet plays a central role in diabetes self-management, allowing individuals to personalize their meal plans based on their preferences, cultural background, lifestyle, and treatment goals. With the help of a registered dietitian or healthcare professional, individuals can learn how different foods affect their blood sugar levels and make appropriate choices to maintain control.

It is important to note that dietary recommendations for diabetes management may vary depending on the individual's type of diabetes, medications, activity level, and other factors. Consulting with a healthcare professional or registered dietitian is highly recommended to develop a personalized and effective diabetes meal plan.

Overview of a diabetes-friendly diet

A diabetes-friendly diet is a healthy eating plan that helps manage blood sugar levels and promotes overall well-being for individuals with diabetes. The primary goal is to maintain stable blood glucose levels by controlling the intake of carbohydrates and making nutritious food choices. Here is an overview of a diabetes-friendly diet:

Carbohydrate Counting: Monitoring carbohydrate intake is crucial for individuals with diabetes. Carbohydrates have the most significant impact on blood sugar levels. The key is to choose high-fiber carbohydrates that digest more slowly, resulting in a gradual rise in blood sugar levels. Whole grains, legumes, fruits, and vegetables are excellent choices.

Portion Control: Keeping portion sizes in check is important to prevent spikes in blood sugar levels. Balancing the quantity of food consumed helps regulate calorie intake, manage weight, and control blood glucose levels. It is advisable to work with a registered dietitian to determine appropriate portion sizes.

Balanced Meals: Creating balanced meals is vital for managing diabetes. A plate method approach is often recommended, where half of the plate consists of non-starchy vegetables such as leafy greens, broccoli, and peppers. One-quarter of the plate can be dedicated to lean proteins like poultry, fish, tofu, or legumes. The remaining quarter can be filled with whole grains or starchy vegetables like sweet potatoes or whole grain bread.

Healthy Fats: Choosing heart-healthy fats is essential for individuals with diabetes. Opt for unsaturated fats found in olive oil, avocados, nuts, and seeds. These fats help improve insulin sensitivity, reduce inflammation, and promote heart health. However, it's important to moderate the consumption of fats as they are high in calories.

Limit Sugar and Processed Foods: It's crucial to limit added sugars and processed foods as they can cause rapid blood sugar spikes. Sugary beverages, sweets, desserts, and processed snacks should be minimized or avoided. Instead, opt for naturally sweetened options like fresh fruits or use artificial sweeteners in moderation, if necessary.

Regular Meal Schedule: Establishing a consistent eating schedule can help regulate blood sugar levels. Spacing out meals and snacks evenly throughout the day prevents extreme fluctuations in glucose levels. It is also important to avoid skipping meals, especially breakfast, as it sets the tone for the day.

Stay Hydrated: Drinking plenty of water is essential for overall health, including diabetes management. It helps maintain hydration, supports metabolism, and aids digestion. Avoid sugary beverages and opt for water, unsweetened tea, or infused water instead.

Individualized Approach: Every person with diabetes is unique, and dietary needs may vary. It's important to work with a registered dietitian or healthcare professional to develop an individualized meal plan that considers personal preferences, cultural factors, medication, and other health conditions.

Remember, a diabetes-friendly diet is just one component of diabetes management. Regular physical activity, monitoring blood sugar levels, taking prescribed medications, and maintaining a healthy weight are also essential for effectively managing diabetes. Consulting with a healthcare team is highly recommended to develop a comprehensive plan tailored to individual needs.

Role of carbohydrates, fats, and proteins

Carbohydrates, fats, and proteins are the three macronutrients that play crucial roles in the human body. Each macronutrient serves specific functions and provides energy in different ways. Here is an overview of the roles of carbohydrates, fats, and proteins:

Carbohydrates

Energy Source: Carbohydrates are the body's primary source of energy. When consumed, they are broken down into glucose, which is used by cells for energy production. Glucose is particularly important for fueling the brain, muscles, and other organs.

Blood Sugar Regulation: Carbohydrates have a significant impact on blood sugar levels. Consuming carbohydrates raises blood glucose levels, triggering the release of insulin from the pancreas to help regulate and transport glucose into cells. This helps maintain stable blood sugar levels.

Fiber and Digestion: Carbohydrates are also a source of dietary fiber, which aids in digestion and promotes bowel regularity. Fiber helps prevent constipation, lowers the risk of heart disease, and assists in maintaining a healthy weight.

Fats

Energy Reserve: Fats are a concentrated source of energy and serve as the body's long-term energy storage. They provide a highly efficient and dense form of energy, supplying fuel during times of calorie deficit or prolonged physical activity.

Protection and Insulation: Fats play a crucial role in protecting vital organs by acting as a cushioning layer. Additionally, they help insulate the body, regulating body temperature and protecting against heat loss.

Nutrient Absorption: Fats are necessary for the absorption of fat-soluble vitamins (vitamins A, D, E, and K). These vitamins require dietary fats to be properly absorbed and utilized by the body.

Proteins

Tissue Building and Repair: Proteins are the building blocks of body tissues, including muscles, organs, skin, hair, and nails. They play a vital role in tissue growth, maintenance, and repair. Proteins are composed of amino acids, which are essential for the synthesis of new proteins in the body.

Enzymes and Hormones: Proteins act as enzymes, facilitating chemical reactions in the body. They also serve as hormones, which regulate various physiological processes and help maintain homeostasis.

Immune Function: Many components of the immune system, including antibodies and immune cells, are made up of proteins. Proteins play a crucial role in defending the body against infections and diseases.

It's important to note that while each macronutrient has its specific role, a balanced diet that includes an appropriate proportion of carbohydrates, fats, and proteins is essential for overall health and well-being. The recommended intake of each macronutrient may vary depending on individual needs, age, sex, physical activity level, and underlying health conditions.

Consulting with a healthcare professional or registered dietitian can help determine the appropriate macronutrient balance for specific dietary requirements.

Key nutrients and their effects on blood sugar levels

Maintaining stable blood sugar levels is important for individuals with diabetes or those looking to manage their overall health. Certain nutrients have varying effects on blood sugar levels. Here are key nutrients and their effects:

Carbohydrates

Impact on Blood Sugar: Carbohydrates have the most significant effect on blood sugar levels as they are broken down into glucose during digestion. Different carbohydrates have varying rates of digestion and absorption, leading to different effects on blood sugar. Simple carbohydrates (e.g., refined sugars) are quickly digested and can cause rapid blood sugar spikes, while complex carbohydrates (e.g., whole grains, legumes, and vegetables) are digested more slowly, resulting in a gradual rise in blood sugar levels.

Recommendations: It is essential to choose high-fiber, complex carbohydrates that have a lower impact on blood sugar levels. These include whole grains, fruits, vegetables, and legumes. Monitoring carbohydrate intake and spreading it out evenly throughout meals can help manage blood sugar levels.

Protein

Impact on Blood Sugar: Protein has a minimal impact on blood sugar levels as it is not directly converted into glucose. However, larger amounts of protein can lead to a modest increase in blood sugar due to a process called gluconeogenesis.

Gluconeogenesis is the conversion of protein into glucose by the liver.

Recommendations: Including lean sources of protein such as poultry, fish, tofu, legumes, and low-fat dairy products in meals can help provide sustained energy and promote satiety without significant effects on blood sugar levels.

Fats

Impact on Blood Sugar: Fats have a minimal impact on blood sugar levels. They are not directly converted into glucose and do not cause significant increases in blood sugar. However, high-fat meals can delay stomach emptying, which may affect the absorption of carbohydrates and impact blood sugar control.

Recommendations: Choosing healthier fats, such as unsaturated fats found in olive oil, avocados, nuts, and seeds, is beneficial for overall health. However, it is important to consume fats in moderation due to their high calorie content.

Fiber

Impact on Blood Sugar: Dietary fiber has a positive effect on blood sugar levels. Soluble fiber, in particular, forms a gel-like substance in the digestive tract, slowing down carbohydrate digestion and absorption. This leads to a more gradual release of glucose into the bloodstream and helps stabilize blood sugar levels.

Recommendations: Including fiber-rich foods, such as whole grains, fruits, vegetables, legumes, and nuts, in the diet is beneficial for managing blood sugar levels. Aim for the recommended daily intake of fiber, which varies depending on age and sex.

Micronutrients (Vitamins and Minerals)

Impact on Blood Sugar: Micronutrients do not have a direct effect on blood sugar levels. However, certain vitamins and minerals play a role in glucose metabolism, insulin sensitivity, and overall metabolic health.

Recommendations: Consuming a varied and balanced diet that includes a wide range of fruits, vegetables, whole grains, lean proteins, and low-fat dairy products helps ensure an adequate intake of essential vitamins and minerals.

It's important to note that individual responses to nutrients may vary, and factors such as portion sizes, meal composition, and individual metabolism can influence blood sugar levels. Monitoring blood sugar regularly and working with a healthcare professional or registered dietitian is crucial for developing a personalized dietary plan that meets specific needs and goals.

Physical activity and exercise

Physical activity and exercise play vital roles in maintaining overall health and well-being. Engaging in regular physical activity offers numerous benefits for both physical and mental health. Here is an overview of physical activity and exercise:

Definition of Physical Activity: Physical activity refers to any bodily movement that requires energy expenditure. It encompasses various daily activities, such as walking, climbing stairs, gardening, housework, and recreational activities.

Definition of Exercise: Exercise is a structured and planned form of physical activity that is performed to improve or maintain physical fitness and overall health. It involves repetitive movements targeting specific muscle groups and is usually performed at a higher intensity than daily activities.

Benefits of Physical Activity and Exercise

Cardiovascular Health: Regular physical activity and exercise improve cardiovascular health by strengthening the heart muscle, improving blood circulation, reducing blood pressure, and lowering the risk of heart disease, stroke, and other cardiovascular conditions.

Weight Management: Physical activity and exercise are important for weight management and preventing obesity. They help burn calories, increase metabolism, and build muscle mass, which can contribute to maintaining a healthy weight or achieving weight loss goals.

Blood Sugar Control: Physical activity and exercise have a positive impact on blood sugar control. They enhance insulin sensitivity, allowing cells to more effectively utilize glucose and regulate blood sugar levels. Regular exercise can be particularly beneficial for individuals with diabetes in managing their condition.

Musculoskeletal Health: Engaging in weight-bearing exercises, such as strength training and resistance exercises, helps build and maintain strong bones, muscles, and joints. This can reduce the risk of osteoporosis, improve bone density, and promote overall musculoskeletal health.

Mental Health and Well-being: Physical activity and exercise have significant mental health benefits. They help reduce symptoms of depression, anxiety, and stress, improve mood, enhance cognitive function, boost self-esteem, and promote better sleep patterns.

Disease Prevention: Regular physical activity and exercise are associated with a reduced risk of chronic diseases such as type 2 diabetes, certain types of cancer (e.g., colon and breast cancer), and metabolic syndrome. They also contribute to better immune function and overall disease resistance.

Improved Energy Levels: Engaging in physical activity and exercise increases energy levels and reduces feelings of fatigue. Regular exercise improves oxygen and nutrient delivery to tissues and enhances overall stamina and endurance.

Longevity and Quality of Life: Numerous studies have shown that individuals who engage in regular physical activity and exercise tend to have a longer lifespan and a higher quality of life. Regular exercise can enhance overall physical function, mobility, and independence, especially in older adults.

It is important to note that individuals should consult with a healthcare professional before starting or significantly changing an exercise regimen, especially if they have underlying health conditions or concerns. The type, intensity, and duration of physical activity should be tailored to individual abilities and goals. Striving for a balanced exercise routine that includes aerobic activities, strength training, flexibility exercises, and rest days is ideal for optimal health benefits.

Types of exercise suitable for individuals with diabetes

Individuals with diabetes can benefit greatly from regular physical activity and exercise. Exercise helps improve insulin sensitivity, regulate blood sugar levels, manage weight, and promote overall health. However, it's important for individuals with diabetes to choose activities that are safe and suitable for their condition. Here are types of exercises that are generally considered suitable for individuals with diabetes:

Aerobic Exercise

Walking: Walking is a low-impact activity that can be easily incorporated into daily routines. It helps improve cardiovascular health, promotes weight management, and aids in blood sugar control.

Cycling: Cycling, whether outdoors or on a stationary bike, is an excellent aerobic exercise that is gentle on the joints. It improves cardiovascular fitness, strengthens leg muscles, and helps burn calories.

Swimming: Swimming and water aerobics provide a full-body workout with minimal impact on joints. They help improve cardiovascular fitness, build muscle strength, and promote flexibility.

Strength Training

Weightlifting: Incorporating weightlifting or resistance training into the exercise routine helps build muscle mass, increase metabolism, and improve insulin sensitivity. It is important to start with light weights and gradually progress under proper guidance.

Bodyweight Exercises: Exercises such as push-ups, squats, lunges, and planks can be performed using one's body weight. They help build strength, improve muscle tone, and enhance overall fitness.

Flexibility and Balance Exercises

Yoga: Yoga combines physical postures, breathing techniques, and meditation. It improves flexibility, balance, and overall mind-body well-being.

Tai Chi: Tai Chi is a gentle form of exercise that focuses on slow, controlled movements, deep breathing, and mindfulness. It helps improve balance, flexibility, and reduces stress.

Interval Training
High-Intensity Interval Training (HIIT): HIIT involves short bursts of intense exercise followed by brief recovery periods. It can be adapted to various activities such as cycling, running, or bodyweight exercises. HIIT improves cardiovascular fitness, enhances insulin sensitivity, and helps burn calories effectively.

Important Considerations
Before starting any exercise program, it is essential to consult with a healthcare professional or a certified exercise specialist, especially if there are pre-existing health conditions or concerns.

Regular monitoring of blood sugar levels before, during, and after exercise is crucial to understand how different activities affect blood glucose levels.

Individuals with diabetes should aim for a minimum of 150 minutes of moderate-intensity aerobic activity per week, spread over at least three days, along with strength training exercises at least twice a week.

It's important to wear comfortable footwear, stay hydrated, and take appropriate precautions to prevent injuries during exercise.

Individuals with diabetes should always carry a source of fast-acting glucose, such as glucose tablets or juice, during exercise in case of low blood sugar episodes (hypoglycemia).

Remember, each person's exercise regimen should be personalized based on individual abilities, preferences, and overall health. Working with healthcare professionals and certified exercise specialists can help develop a safe and effective exercise plan tailored to specific needs and goals.

Incorporating physical activity into daily routine

Incorporating physical activity into your daily routine is an effective way to maintain an active lifestyle and reap the health benefits of regular exercise. Here are some tips to help you integrate physical activity into your day-to-day life:

Prioritize Movement: Make physical activity a priority and view it as an essential part of your daily routine. Set aside dedicated time for exercise and treat it as a non-negotiable appointment with yourself.

Set Realistic Goals: Start by setting realistic and achievable goals for physical activity. Begin with small steps and gradually increase the duration and intensity of your activities over time. This approach helps build consistency and prevents burnout or injury.

Active Commuting: If possible, consider incorporating active modes of transportation into your daily commute. Walk or bike to work or public transportation stations instead of driving. If your commute is long, try getting off a few stops earlier and walking the remaining distance.

Take Breaks and Move Regularly: Break up long periods of sitting or sedentary work by taking short movement breaks. Set a reminder to stand up, stretch, or walk around every hour. Consider using a standing desk or incorporating active sitting options, such as a stability ball or adjustable desk chair.

Walk Whenever Possible: Walking is a simple and accessible form of physical activity. Whenever possible, choose to walk instead of driving for short distances. Take a brisk walk during your lunch break or after dinner. Use stairs instead of elevators whenever feasible.

Make Chores Active: Turn household chores into opportunities for physical activity. Vacuuming, mopping, gardening, and cleaning can provide a workout for your muscles. Put on some music and make it enjoyable.

Schedule Active Breaks at Work: If you have a sedentary job, find ways to incorporate movement into your workday. Take short walks during breaks, use standing or adjustable desks, or engage in desk exercises, such as stretching or leg lifts.

Involve Friends and Family: Make physical activity a social event by involving friends or family members. Take walks or bike rides together, participate in group exercise classes, or join sports teams or recreational activities as a group.

Utilize Technology: Use fitness apps, activity trackers, or smartwatches to monitor your daily steps, track workouts, and set reminders for physical activity. These tools can provide motivation and help you stay accountable.

Find Activities You Enjoy: Engaging in physical activities that you enjoy increases the likelihood of sticking with them. Explore different activities such as dancing, swimming, hiking, or team sports to find what resonates with you.

Remember, the key is to find opportunities to move more throughout the day and make physical activity a regular part of your lifestyle. By incorporating physical activity into your daily routine, you can experience the numerous health benefits and improve your overall well-being.

Weight management and its impact on diabetes

Weight management plays a crucial role in the management and prevention of diabetes. Maintaining a healthy weight can have a significant impact on blood sugar control, insulin sensitivity, and overall health for individuals with diabetes. Here are the ways in which weight management can positively affect diabetes:

Improved Insulin Sensitivity: Excess weight, particularly abdominal or visceral fat, can contribute to insulin resistance, where the body's cells become less responsive to insulin. This leads to elevated blood sugar levels. Losing weight and reducing body fat can improve insulin sensitivity, allowing the body to utilize insulin more effectively and regulate blood sugar levels.

Blood Sugar Control: Weight management, especially through a combination of healthy eating and regular physical activity, can help stabilize blood sugar levels. By achieving and maintaining a healthy weight, individuals with diabetes may require fewer diabetes medications or insulin, as their bodies become more efficient at utilizing glucose.

Reduced Risk of Type 2 Diabetes: Obesity and excess weight are significant risk factors for developing type 2 diabetes. Engaging in weight management efforts, such as losing weight and maintaining a healthy weight, can lower the risk of developing type 2 diabetes in high-risk individuals, such as those with prediabetes or a family history of the disease.

Cardiovascular Health: Weight management has a positive impact on cardiovascular health, which is crucial for individuals with diabetes who are at an increased risk of heart disease and stroke. Losing weight can help lower blood pressure, reduce LDL (bad) cholesterol levels, and improve overall lipid profile, thus reducing the risk of cardiovascular complications.

Increased Energy and Physical Function: Maintaining a healthy weight can lead to increased energy levels and improved physical function. Losing excess weight can alleviate the strain on joints, improve mobility, and enhance overall quality of life for individuals with diabetes.

Overall Health Benefits: Weight management has broader health benefits beyond diabetes management. It can help prevent or manage other obesity-related conditions, such as sleep apnea, certain types of cancer, fatty liver disease, and joint problems. Achieving a healthy weight promotes overall well-being and reduces the risk of various chronic diseases.

It is important to approach weight management in a holistic and sustainable manner. This includes adopting a balanced and nutritious eating plan, engaging in regular physical activity, managing stress levels, getting adequate sleep, and seeking support from healthcare professionals, such as registered dietitians and certified diabetes educators.

Individuals with diabetes should work with their healthcare team to develop a personalized weight management plan that takes into account their specific health needs, medication adjustments, and blood sugar monitoring. Slow and steady weight loss, aiming for a weight loss of 1-2 pounds per week, is generally recommended for long-term success and improved health outcomes.

Strategies for achieving and maintaining a healthy weight

Achieving and maintaining a healthy weight is a multifaceted process that involves making sustainable lifestyle changes. Here are some strategies to help you achieve and maintain a healthy weight:

1. Set Realistic Goals: Set achievable and realistic goals for weight loss or weight maintenance. Aim for gradual and sustainable changes rather than quick fixes. Consult with a healthcare professional or registered dietitian to determine an appropriate weight loss goal based on your individual needs and health status.

2. Adopt a Balanced Eating Plan:
   - Choose Nutrient-Dense Foods: Focus on consuming foods that are rich in nutrients and lower in calories. Include plenty of fruits, vegetables, whole grains, lean proteins, and healthy fats in your diet.

- Practice Portion Control: Be mindful of portion sizes and avoid oversized servings. Use smaller plates, bowls, and cups to help control portions.

- Practice Mindful Eating: Pay attention to hunger and fullness cues, eat slowly, and savor each bite. Avoid distractions such as television or electronic devices while eating.

- Limit Processed Foods and Sugary Drinks: Minimize the intake of processed foods, sugary snacks, sodas, and sugary beverages, as they are often high in calories and low in nutrients.

3. Regular Physical Activity:

- Incorporate Aerobic Exercises: Engage in moderate-intensity aerobic exercises such as brisk walking, cycling, swimming, or dancing for at least 150 minutes per week. Gradually increase the duration and intensity of your workouts.

- Include Strength Training: Include strength training exercises at least two days a week to build lean muscle mass.

Resistance training can help boost metabolism and improve body composition.

- Be Active Throughout the Day: Look for opportunities to increase your daily activity level. Take the stairs instead of the elevator, walk or bike to nearby destinations, and take breaks to stretch or walk during sedentary periods.

4. Practice Healthy Eating Habits:

- Eat Regularly: Establish regular eating patterns by having balanced meals and snacks at consistent times throughout the day. This can help prevent overeating and stabilize blood sugar levels.

- Control Emotional Eating: Identify and find alternative coping mechanisms for emotional eating triggers. Seek support from friends, family, or professionals if needed.

- Keep a Food Diary: Track your food intake to increase awareness of eating patterns and identify areas for improvement. It can help you make informed choices and hold yourself accountable.

5. Get Adequate Sleep: Prioritize getting enough sleep as it plays a role in weight management. Aim for 7-9 hours of quality sleep per night. Poor sleep can disrupt hunger hormones and lead to increased food cravings and weight gain.

6. Manage Stress: Find healthy ways to manage stress as it can contribute to emotional eating and weight gain. Practice stress-reducing techniques such as exercise, meditation, deep breathing, or engaging in hobbies and activities you enjoy.

7. Seek Support: Engage the support of healthcare professionals, such as registered dietitians or certified diabetes educators, who can provide personalized guidance and support throughout your weight management journey. Consider joining

support groups or seeking help from friends and family to stay motivated.

Remember, achieving and maintaining a healthy weight is a long-term commitment. It's important to make sustainable lifestyle changes rather than pursuing short-term solutions. Focus on overall health and well-being rather than solely on the number on the scale. Be patient, persistent, and kind to yourself as you work towards your weight management goals.

Understanding the link between obesity and diabetes

Obesity and diabetes are closely interconnected, with obesity being a significant risk factor for the development of type 2 diabetes. Understanding the link between obesity and diabetes is crucial for prevention, management, and overall health. Here are some key points to consider:

1. Insulin Resistance: Obesity is often associated with a condition called insulin resistance, where the body's cells become less responsive to the hormone insulin. Insulin is responsible for regulating blood sugar levels by allowing glucose to enter cells to be used as energy. In individuals with insulin resistance, the pancreas produces more insulin to compensate, but the cells do not respond appropriately, leading to elevated blood sugar levels and potentially the development of type 2 diabetes.

2. Adipose Tissue and Inflammation: Excess body fat, especially abdominal or visceral fat, is metabolically active and releases various substances that can contribute to inflammation. Chronic low-grade inflammation is thought to play a role in insulin resistance and the development of type 2 diabetes.

3. Hormonal Imbalances: Adipose tissue, particularly visceral fat, can release hormones and signaling molecules that can disrupt the normal balance of hormones involved in glucose metabolism, such as adipokines, leptin, and resistin. These imbalances can further contribute to insulin resistance and diabetes.

4. Increased Fat Storage: Obesity often leads to an increase in the storage of fat in tissues other than adipose tissue, such as the liver, muscles, and pancreas. Fat accumulation in these organs can interfere with their normal functioning and contribute to insulin resistance and impaired glucose regulation.

5. Metabolic Syndrome: Obesity is a major component of metabolic syndrome, a cluster of conditions that includes abdominal obesity, high blood pressure, high blood sugar levels, and abnormal cholesterol levels. People with metabolic syndrome are

at a significantly higher risk of developing type 2 diabetes.

6. Impact on Beta Cells: Obesity and excess body fat can place increased demands on the insulin-producing beta cells in the pancreas. Over time, the beta cells may struggle to keep up with the insulin demands, leading to a decline in insulin production and secretion, further contributing to the development of type 2 diabetes.

7. Vicious Cycle: Obesity and diabetes can create a vicious cycle. Excess weight increases the risk of developing diabetes, and once diabetes is present, the elevated blood sugar levels can further promote weight gain and difficulty in losing weight.

It's important to note that while obesity is a significant risk factor, not all individuals with obesity develop diabetes, and not all individuals with diabetes are obese. Genetic factors, lifestyle choices, diet, physical activity levels, and other individual factors also play a role in the development of diabetes.

Prevention and management of obesity can help reduce the risk of developing type 2 diabetes. Promoting a healthy lifestyle that includes a balanced diet, regular physical activity, weight management, and overall wellness is essential. If you have concerns about your weight or risk of diabetes, it's recommended to consult with a healthcare professional for personalized guidance, screening, and support.

3

Blood Sugar Control

Blood sugar control, also known as glucose control, is a fundamental aspect of managing diabetes and promoting overall health. It involves maintaining blood sugar levels within a target range to prevent complications and ensure optimal functioning of the body. Here are key points to understand about blood sugar control:

1. Monitoring Blood Sugar Levels: Regular monitoring of blood sugar levels is crucial for understanding how your body responds to food, physical activity, medication, and other factors. This is typically done using a blood glucose meter or continuous glucose monitoring (CGM) devices. Monitoring helps identify patterns, make informed decisions, and adjust treatment plans as needed.

2. Medications and Insulin: Depending on the type and severity of diabetes, medication or insulin therapy may be prescribed to help control blood sugar levels. These medications work by either increasing insulin production, improving insulin sensitivity, slowing down glucose absorption, or reducing glucose production by the liver. It is important to take prescribed medications as directed by healthcare professionals.

3. Healthy Eating Plan: A balanced and individualized meal plan is essential for blood sugar control. Focus on consuming a variety of nutrient-dense foods, including whole grains, lean proteins, fruits, vegetables, and healthy fats. Portion control, carbohydrate counting, and spacing meals evenly throughout the day can help maintain steady blood sugar levels.

4. Carbohydrate Management: Carbohydrates have the most significant impact on blood sugar levels. Understanding how different carbohydrates affect blood sugar and learning to manage their intake is essential. Consistency in carbohydrate intake, portion sizes, and considering the glycemic index of foods can help maintain stable blood sugar levels.

5. Physical Activity: Regular physical activity has a positive impact on blood sugar control. Exercise increases insulin sensitivity, allowing glucose to enter cells more effectively, which can lower blood sugar levels. Engaging in aerobic exercises, strength training, and incorporating physical activity into daily routines are beneficial. However, it is important to monitor blood sugar levels during and after exercise to prevent hypoglycemia or hyperglycemia.

6. Stress Management: Stress can affect blood sugar levels by triggering hormonal responses that raise glucose levels. Managing stress through relaxation techniques, regular exercise, mindfulness, and seeking support can help promote better blood sugar control.

7. Adequate Sleep: Poor sleep or inadequate sleep can disrupt blood sugar regulation. Aim for 7-9 hours of quality sleep each night to support optimal blood sugar control and overall health.

8. Regular Healthcare Follow-ups: Regular visits to healthcare professionals, such as doctors, diabetes educators, and registered dietitians, are important for ongoing management of blood sugar control. They can provide guidance, monitor progress, adjust medications if necessary, and help address any concerns or challenges.

9. Education and Self-Management: Educating yourself about diabetes management, blood sugar control, and healthy lifestyle choices is empowering. Learning how to interpret blood sugar readings, understand the effects of food and exercise, and recognize signs of hypo- or hyperglycemia enables better self-management.

10. Support System: Having a support system, whether it's family, friends, or support groups, can make a significant difference in managing blood sugar control. Sharing experiences, exchanging tips, and receiving encouragement can help individuals stay motivated and committed to their diabetes management goals.

Remember, blood sugar control is a personalized journey, and the target ranges may vary depending on individual factors and healthcare recommendations. Working closely with healthcare professionals and making necessary adjustments based on regular monitoring is key to achieving optimal blood sugar control and maintaining overall well-being.

Monitoring blood glucose levels

Monitoring blood glucose levels is an essential part of diabetes management. It allows individuals to understand their blood sugar patterns, make informed decisions regarding medication, lifestyle choices, and adjustments to their diabetes management plan. Here are key points to understand about monitoring blood glucose levels:

1. Blood Glucose Meters: Blood glucose meters are commonly used for self-monitoring of blood glucose levels. These portable devices require a small blood sample obtained by pricking the fingertip with a lancet. The blood sample is then applied to a test strip inserted into the meter, which provides a blood glucose reading within seconds.

2. Continuous Glucose Monitoring (CGM) Systems: CGM systems are devices that continuously measure glucose levels throughout the day and night. They consist of a small sensor inserted under the skin, usually on the abdomen or arm, that measures glucose levels in the interstitial fluid. The sensor sends real-time glucose readings to a receiver or smartphone app, allowing individuals to monitor their glucose levels continuously.

3. Frequency of Monitoring: The frequency of blood glucose monitoring may vary depending on factors such as diabetes type, treatment plan, medication, and individual needs. Some individuals may need to monitor multiple times a day, while others may require less frequent monitoring. Healthcare professionals can provide personalized recommendations for monitoring frequency.

4. Timing of Blood Glucose Checks: It's important to monitor blood glucose levels at different times to gain a comprehensive understanding of how blood sugar responds to various factors. Common times for monitoring include before meals (preprandial), after meals (postprandial), before bedtime, and occasionally during the night.

5. Target Range: Each individual may have a specific target range for blood glucose levels based on their diabetes type, age, overall health, and treatment goals. Target ranges may be different for fasting blood sugar, pre- and post-meal levels, and bedtime readings. Healthcare professionals can help determine the appropriate target range for each person.

6. Record Keeping: Keeping a record of blood glucose readings is valuable for tracking trends, identifying patterns, and sharing information with healthcare

professionals. This can be done using paper logs, digital applications, or online platforms specifically designed for diabetes management.

7. Hypoglycemia (Low Blood Sugar) and Hyperglycemia (High Blood Sugar): Monitoring blood glucose levels helps detect episodes of hypoglycemia (blood sugar below target range) and hyperglycemia (blood sugar above target range). Prompt action can be taken to treat low blood sugar with fast-acting carbohydrates and prevent complications associated with high blood sugar.

8. Adjusting Treatment Plan: Blood glucose monitoring provides valuable information for adjusting diabetes management plans. If blood sugar levels consistently fall outside the target range, healthcare professionals may recommend adjustments in medication, diet, physical activity, or other aspects of the treatment plan.

9. Education and Support: It's important to receive proper education on using blood glucose monitoring devices, interpreting results, and understanding the factors that can affect blood sugar levels. Diabetes educators, healthcare professionals, and support groups can provide guidance, answer questions, and offer support in the monitoring process.

Regular blood glucose monitoring empowers individuals to take an active role in their diabetes management and make informed decisions to maintain optimal blood sugar control. It is essential to work closely with healthcare professionals to develop an individualized monitoring plan and use the results to guide effective diabetes management.

Importance of regular monitoring

Regular monitoring of blood sugar levels is crucial for individuals with diabetes. Here are some key reasons highlighting the importance of regular blood sugar monitoring:

1. Diabetes Management: Blood sugar monitoring is a vital component of diabetes management. It provides valuable information about how the body is responding to medications, lifestyle choices, and other factors. By monitoring blood sugar levels, individuals can make informed decisions regarding their treatment plan, including medication adjustments, dietary modifications, and exercise routines.

2. Glycemic Control: Monitoring blood sugar levels helps individuals achieve and maintain glycemic control. This means keeping blood sugar levels within a target range recommended by healthcare professionals. Maintaining stable blood sugar levels can prevent short-term complications such as hyperglycemia (high blood sugar) or hypoglycemia (low blood

sugar) and reduce the risk of long-term complications associated with diabetes.

3. Individualized Treatment: Every person with diabetes is unique, and blood sugar levels can vary significantly between individuals. Regular monitoring allows for personalized treatment plans tailored to individual needs. By understanding one's blood sugar patterns, healthcare professionals can make appropriate recommendations for medication, lifestyle modifications, and other interventions.

4. Adjusting Medications: Blood sugar monitoring provides essential information for adjusting diabetes medications. It helps determine if current medications are effectively managing blood sugar levels or if adjustments are necessary. This includes oral medications, insulin, and other injectable diabetes medications. Timely medication adjustments based on blood

sugar readings can help maintain optimal glycemic control.

5. Identifying Patterns and Trends: Regular blood sugar monitoring helps identify patterns and trends in blood sugar levels. By tracking levels before and after meals, at different times of the day, or in response to specific activities, individuals can identify factors that affect their blood sugar. This insight enables them to make informed choices about diet, exercise, stress management, and other lifestyle factors that can impact blood sugar control.

6. Hypoglycemia and Hyperglycemia Detection: Blood sugar monitoring helps detect episodes of hypoglycemia (low blood sugar) and hyperglycemia (high blood sugar). Hypoglycemia can be dangerous and requires immediate treatment to prevent complications. On the other hand, uncontrolled hyperglycemia can lead to long-term complications such as nerve

damage, kidney problems, and cardiovascular issues. Regular monitoring helps individuals take timely action to prevent or manage these episodes.

7. Diabetes Self-Management: Regular blood sugar monitoring empowers individuals to take an active role in their diabetes self-management. By understanding how their choices impact blood sugar levels, individuals can make adjustments to their diet, exercise, stress management, and medication use. It promotes self-awareness, accountability, and a sense of control over one's diabetes management.

8. Communication with Healthcare Professionals: Blood sugar readings provide valuable information that can be shared with healthcare professionals during regular check-ups or appointments. By reviewing blood sugar data, healthcare professionals can assess treatment effectiveness, make

appropriate adjustments, and provide personalized guidance and support.

Remember, regular blood sugar monitoring should be done in conjunction with guidance from healthcare professionals. They can provide specific recommendations regarding the frequency of monitoring, target ranges, and interpretation of results based on individual circumstances. By actively monitoring blood sugar levels, individuals can optimize their diabetes management and improve overall health outcomes.

Techniques for accurate measurement

To ensure accurate measurement of blood sugar levels, it is important to follow proper techniques when using a blood glucose meter. Here are some techniques to help achieve accurate measurements:

1. Clean Hands: Wash your hands thoroughly with warm water and soap before testing your blood sugar. This helps remove any dirt, food residue, or substances that could affect the accuracy of the reading.

2. Use New Lancets and Test Strips: Always use a new lancet (the small needle used to prick the fingertip) for each blood sugar test to ensure a clean and sharp puncture. Similarly, use fresh, unexpired test strips that are specifically designed for your blood glucose meter.

3. Calibrate the Meter: If your blood glucose meter requires calibration, follow the instructions provided by the manufacturer to ensure accurate readings. This usually involves inserting a calibration code or scanning a code with the meter.

4. Fingerstick Technique: Choose a clean and dry fingertip, preferably on the side of the finger rather than the pad. Use a lancet

device to obtain a small drop of blood. Avoid squeezing the finger excessively, as this may distort the blood sample and lead to inaccurate results.

5. Apply Blood Correctly: Apply the blood sample to the designated area on the test strip according to the instructions provided with your blood glucose meter. Ensure that an adequate amount of blood is applied to the strip for an accurate reading. Avoid applying blood to the top or bottom edge of the strip.

6. Proper Storage of Test Strips: Store your test strips according to the manufacturer's instructions, typically in a cool, dry place, away from extreme temperatures and humidity. Exposure to moisture or extreme conditions may affect the accuracy of the test strips.

7. Control Solution: Regularly check the accuracy of your blood glucose meter using

a control solution provided by the manufacturer. This solution contains a known glucose concentration that allows you to verify if your meter is providing accurate readings.

8. Monitor Meter Performance: Keep an eye on the performance of your blood glucose meter. If you notice significant discrepancies between meter readings and how you feel, or if you suspect the meter may be malfunctioning, contact the manufacturer or your healthcare professional for assistance.

9. Periodic Meter Maintenance: Follow the maintenance instructions provided by the manufacturer to keep your blood glucose meter in good working condition. This may include cleaning the meter, ensuring the battery is properly charged or replaced, and conducting any recommended maintenance procedures.

10. Regular Meter Verification: Periodically compare your blood glucose meter readings with those obtained from laboratory tests. This helps ensure the accuracy and reliability of your meter. Discuss any significant discrepancies with your healthcare professional.

Remember, accurate measurement of blood sugar levels is essential for effective diabetes management. Following these techniques and using your blood glucose meter correctly can help you obtain reliable readings and make informed decisions regarding your diabetes treatment plan. If you have any concerns about the accuracy of your blood glucose meter or your blood sugar control, consult with your healthcare professional for guidance and support.

Medications and insulin therapy

Medications and insulin therapy play a crucial role in the management of diabetes, particularly for individuals with type 1 diabetes and some individuals with type 2 diabetes. These medications are prescribed by healthcare professionals to help control blood sugar levels and prevent complications. Here are some common medications and insulin therapy options used in the treatment of diabetes:

1. Insulin: Insulin is a hormone that regulates blood sugar levels by facilitating the uptake of glucose from the bloodstream into cells. People with type 1 diabetes, and some with type 2 diabetes, require insulin therapy because their bodies either do not produce insulin (type 1) or do not use it effectively (type 2). Insulin is typically administered through injections or insulin pump devices. There are several types of insulin, including:

   - Rapid-acting insulin: Starts working within 15 minutes, peaks in about 1 hour, and lasts for 2 to 4 hours.

- Short-acting insulin: Begins working within 30 minutes, peaks in 2 to 3 hours, and lasts for about 6 to 8 hours.
- Intermediate-acting insulin: Takes effect within 1 to 2 hours, peaks in 4 to 6 hours, and lasts for about 12 to 16 hours.
- Long-acting insulin: Works gradually and consistently over an extended period, typically lasting 24 hours or more.

2. Oral Medications for Type 2 Diabetes: For individuals with type 2 diabetes, oral medications may be prescribed to help manage blood sugar levels. These medications work in various ways, including:

- Metformin: Reduces glucose production in the liver, improves insulin sensitivity, and enhances glucose uptake by cells.
- Sulfonylureas: Stimulate the pancreas to release more insulin.
- Thiazolidinediones: Increase insulin sensitivity and improve glucose utilization.

- Dipeptidyl peptidase-4 (DPP-4) inhibitors: Increase insulin release and reduce glucagon secretion.

- Sodium-glucose cotransporter-2 (SGLT2) inhibitors: Lower blood sugar levels by increasing the excretion of glucose through urine.

3. GLP-1 Receptor Agonists: GLP-1 receptor agonists are injectable medications used for type 2 diabetes. They work by stimulating insulin secretion, reducing glucagon production, slowing down gastric emptying, and promoting a feeling of fullness. These medications are typically taken once or twice daily or as weekly injections.

4. Combination Therapy: In some cases, healthcare professionals may prescribe a combination of oral medications, injectable medications, and/or insulin therapy to achieve optimal blood sugar control. This approach allows for targeting multiple

aspects of diabetes management and tailoring treatment to individual needs.

It's important to note that the specific medications and insulin therapy options prescribed may vary depending on various factors, such as the type of diabetes, individual health needs, other medical conditions, and personal preferences. The dosage and timing of medications or insulin therapy are determined by healthcare professionals based on individual requirements.

It is crucial to work closely with healthcare professionals, such as doctors, diabetes educators, or endocrinologists, to understand the medications or insulin therapy prescribed, receive proper instructions for administration, and monitor for any potential side effects or complications. Regular communication and follow-up appointments are important to ensure that the treatment plan is effective and adjusted as necessary for optimal blood sugar control.

Overview of common diabetes medications

Here is an overview of some common medications used in the management of diabetes:

1. Metformin: Metformin is often the first-line medication for type 2 diabetes. It works by reducing glucose production in the liver and improving insulin sensitivity, allowing cells to better utilize glucose. Metformin may also help with weight management and has shown benefits in reducing the risk of cardiovascular complications.

2. Sulfonylureas: Sulfonylureas stimulate the release of insulin from the pancreas. They help lower blood sugar levels by increasing insulin production. Examples of

sulfonylureas include glimepiride, glipizide, and glyburide. These medications are usually taken orally.

3. Meglitinides: Meglitinides, such as repaglinide and nateglinide, also stimulate insulin release from the pancreas, but their effect is shorter-acting compared to sulfonylureas. They are taken orally before meals to help control post-meal blood sugar spikes.

4. Thiazolidinediones: Thiazolidinediones, or TZDs, improve insulin sensitivity and reduce insulin resistance. They help the body use insulin more effectively. Examples of TZDs include pioglitazone and rosiglitazone. These medications are taken orally.

5. Dipeptidyl Peptidase-4 (DPP-4) Inhibitors: DPP-4 inhibitors, such as sitagliptin, saxagliptin, and linagliptin, increase the levels of incretin hormones in

the body. These hormones help stimulate insulin release and reduce glucagon secretion, resulting in lower blood sugar levels. DPP-4 inhibitors are taken orally.

6. Sodium-Glucose Cotransporter-2 (SGLT2) Inhibitors: SGLT2 inhibitors, including canagliflozin, dapagliflozin, and empagliflozin, work by blocking the reabsorption of glucose in the kidneys, leading to increased glucose excretion through urine. They can help lower blood sugar levels and may also have benefits for blood pressure and weight management.

7. GLP-1 Receptor Agonists: GLP-1 receptor agonists, such as exenatide, liraglutide, and dulaglutide, mimic the action of incretin hormones. They stimulate insulin release, suppress glucagon secretion, slow down gastric emptying, and promote a feeling of fullness. GLP-1 receptor agonists are usually administered through injection and are

available in both short-acting and long-acting formulations.

8. Insulin: Insulin therapy is essential for individuals with type 1 diabetes and may be prescribed for some with type 2 diabetes who cannot achieve adequate blood sugar control with oral medications alone. Insulin is available in different types, including rapid-acting, short-acting, intermediate-acting, and long-acting formulations. Insulin can be injected using a syringe, insulin pen, or insulin pump.

It's important to note that the choice of medication depends on several factors, including the type of diabetes, individual health needs, other medical conditions, and potential side effects. The dosage and combination of medications will be determined by healthcare professionals based on individual circumstances and ongoing monitoring of blood sugar levels.

Diabetes medications are typically prescribed in conjunction with lifestyle modifications, such as a healthy diet, regular physical activity, and weight management, to achieve optimal blood sugar control and reduce the risk of complications. It is essential to work closely with healthcare professionals to understand the medications prescribed, adhere to the treatment plan, and regularly monitor blood sugar levels.

Insulin therapy and its role in managing diabetes

Insulin therapy plays a critical role in managing diabetes, particularly for individuals with type 1 diabetes and some individuals with type 2 diabetes. Insulin is a hormone produced by the pancreas that helps regulate blood sugar levels. In people with diabetes, either the body does not produce insulin (type 1) or does not use it effectively (type 2), leading to elevated blood sugar levels. Insulin therapy aims to restore normal insulin levels and maintain optimal blood sugar control. Here are some key aspects of insulin therapy and its role in managing diabetes:

1. Type 1 Diabetes: Individuals with type 1 diabetes have an absolute deficiency of insulin and therefore require insulin therapy to survive. Insulin is administered through injections or insulin pump devices to mimic the normal release of insulin by the pancreas. Multiple daily injections or continuous subcutaneous insulin infusion (insulin pump) are used to provide basal (background) insulin levels and bolus (mealtime) insulin doses to cover carbohydrate intake. This helps regulate blood sugar levels and prevent complications associated with high blood sugar.

2. Type 2 Diabetes: In type 2 diabetes, insulin therapy may be prescribed when other oral medications or lifestyle

modifications are insufficient to achieve target blood sugar levels. It is often used as an adjunct to oral medications. Insulin therapy can help improve blood sugar control by providing additional insulin to overcome insulin resistance or improve the pancreas' ability to produce insulin. The type and timing of insulin used will depend on individual needs and treatment goals.

3. Insulin Types: Insulin therapy includes different types of insulin that vary in their onset, peak, and duration of action. These types include:

- Rapid-Acting Insulin: It begins to work within 15 minutes, reaches its peak effect in about 1 hour, and lasts for 2 to 4 hours. Rapid-acting insulin is typically taken before meals to cover the rise in blood sugar after eating.

- Short-Acting Insulin: It starts working within 30 minutes, peaks in 2 to 3 hours, and lasts for about 6 to 8 hours. Short-acting insulin is usually taken before meals to cover blood sugar elevation during that time.

- Intermediate-Acting Insulin: It takes effect within 1 to 2 hours, peaks in 4 to 6 hours, and lasts for about 12 to 16 hours. Intermediate-acting insulin provides basal insulin coverage and helps maintain stable blood sugar levels between meals and overnight.

- Long-Acting Insulin: It works gradually and consistently over an extended period, typically lasting 24 hours or more. Long-acting insulin provides basal insulin coverage without pronounced peaks and helps maintain blood sugar stability throughout the day.

4. Insulin Administration: Insulin can be administered through various methods, including:

- Injections: Insulin is injected subcutaneously (into the fatty tissue just below the skin) using a syringe, insulin pen, or insulin pen needle. Injections are usually self-administered by individuals with diabetes or their caregivers.

- Insulin Pumps: Insulin pumps are small devices that deliver insulin continuously through a catheter inserted under the skin. They provide both basal and bolus insulin doses and allow for more precise insulin delivery. Insulin pumps require regular monitoring and programming to ensure appropriate insulin delivery.

5. Individualized Treatment: Insulin therapy is highly individualized to meet the specific needs of each person with diabetes. Factors such as age, weight, lifestyle, blood sugar control goals, and personal preferences are taken into account when determining the appropriate type and dosage of insulin. Healthcare professionals work closely with

individuals to develop an insulin regimen that fits their lifestyle and ensures optimal blood sugar control.

6. Blood Sugar Monitoring: Regular blood sugar monitoring is

 essential for individuals on insulin therapy to adjust insulin doses, prevent hypoglycemia (low blood sugar), and optimize blood sugar control. Self-monitoring of blood glucose levels helps individuals make informed decisions about insulin administration, diet, and physical activity.

Insulin therapy plays a vital role in managing diabetes by helping to regulate blood sugar levels and prevent acute and long-term complications. It is important for individuals on insulin therapy to work closely with healthcare professionals, including doctors, diabetes educators, or endocrinologists, to receive proper insulin dosage guidance, learn appropriate injection techniques, and monitor for any potential side effects or complications. Regular communication and follow-up appointments are crucial to ensure that the insulin regimen is tailored to individual needs and adjusted as necessary for optimal blood sugar control.

Alternative therapies and complementary approaches

In addition to conventional medical treatments, some individuals with diabetes may explore alternative therapies and complementary approaches to manage their condition. It's important to note that while these therapies may offer additional support, they should not replace or be used as a substitute for standard medical care. Here are some alternative therapies and complementary approaches that are sometimes considered:

1. Herbal and Nutritional Supplements: Certain herbs and nutritional supplements have been studied for their potential benefits in managing blood sugar levels. Examples include:

- Cinnamon: Some studies suggest that cinnamon may have a modest effect in lowering blood sugar levels, but further research is needed to establish its effectiveness.

- Chromium: Chromium is a mineral that has been investigated for its potential role in improving insulin sensitivity. However, the evidence is inconclusive, and supplementation should be approached with caution.

- Alpha-Lipoic Acid: Alpha-lipoic acid is an antioxidant that has shown promise in reducing nerve damage related to diabetes. It may also help improve insulin sensitivity, but more research is needed.

It's important to consult with a healthcare professional before starting any herbal or nutritional supplement, as they can interact with medications or have adverse effects.

2. Acupuncture: Acupuncture is an ancient Chinese practice that involves inserting thin needles into specific points on the body. Some studies suggest that acupuncture may help improve blood sugar control and alleviate diabetic neuropathy symptoms. However, more research is needed to establish its effectiveness in managing diabetes.

3. Mind-Body Techniques: Stress management techniques, such as meditation, yoga, and deep breathing exercises, may help individuals with diabetes better manage their condition. These techniques can promote relaxation, reduce stress, and improve overall well-being.

4. Massage Therapy: Massage therapy may help improve circulation, reduce muscle tension, and promote relaxation. While it may provide temporary relief from certain diabetes-related symptoms, such as neuropathy or muscle stiffness, it does not directly treat the underlying condition.

5. Chiropractic Care: Chiropractic care focuses on spinal alignment and nervous system function. Some individuals with diabetes seek chiropractic treatments to alleviate neuropathy symptoms or improve overall wellness. However, evidence supporting its effectiveness in managing diabetes is limited.

6. Exercise and Physical Activity: Regular exercise is not considered an alternative therapy, but it is an important complement to standard diabetes management. Physical activity can help improve insulin sensitivity, lower blood sugar levels, manage weight, and enhance overall cardiovascular health.

It is recommended to engage in a combination of aerobic exercises (e.g., walking, swimming) and strength training.

It is crucial to discuss any alternative therapies or complementary approaches with a healthcare professional. They can provide guidance, evaluate the safety and potential interactions, and help integrate them into an individual's comprehensive diabetes management plan. Additionally, it's important to continue regular medical check-ups and adhere to prescribed medications and lifestyle modifications.

Herbal remedies and supplements

Herbal remedies and supplements are often sought as alternative or complementary approaches to managing diabetes. While some herbs and supplements may have potential benefits, it's important to note that they should not replace or be used as a substitute for standard medical care. If considering the use of herbal remedies or supplements, it's crucial to consult with a healthcare professional to ensure their safety and effectiveness, as well as potential interactions with medications. Here are some commonly mentioned herbs and supplements for diabetes:

1. Cinnamon: Cinnamon has been studied for its potential to improve blood sugar control. Some research suggests that cinnamon may help lower fasting blood sugar levels and improve insulin sensitivity. However, the evidence is limited, and more studies are needed to establish its effectiveness and determine the appropriate dosage.

2. Chromium: Chromium is a mineral that has been investigated for its role in blood sugar metabolism. It is involved in the action of insulin and may help improve insulin sensitivity. However, the evidence regarding its effectiveness in diabetes

management is inconclusive, and supplementation should be approached with caution.

3. Alpha-Lipoic Acid (ALA): Alpha-lipoic acid is an antioxidant that may have benefits for individuals with diabetes. It has been studied for its potential to reduce nerve damage (diabetic neuropathy) and improve insulin sensitivity. ALA may also help reduce oxidative stress associated with diabetes. However, further research is needed to establish its efficacy and determine the appropriate dosage.

4. Ginseng: Ginseng is a traditional herb that has been used in traditional medicine for various purposes, including blood sugar control. Some studies suggest that certain types of ginseng, such as American ginseng and Korean red ginseng, may help improve blood sugar control and enhance insulin sensitivity. However, more research is

needed to confirm these effects and determine optimal dosages.

5. Bitter Melon: Bitter melon, a vegetable commonly used in Asian cuisine, has been studied for its potential antidiabetic effects. It may help lower blood sugar levels by increasing insulin secretion and improving glucose uptake. However, evidence regarding its effectiveness in diabetes management is limited, and it may cause gastrointestinal side effects.

6. Gymnema Sylvestre: Gymnema sylvestre is an herb traditionally used in Ayurvedic medicine for its potential to regulate blood sugar levels. It may help reduce sugar cravings, lower blood sugar levels, and improve insulin secretion. However, more research is needed to establish its effectiveness and determine the appropriate dosage.

It is important to approach herbal remedies and supplements with caution. Their safety, efficacy, and appropriate dosage can vary, and they may have interactions with medications or cause adverse effects. It is always recommended to consult with a healthcare professional before starting any herbal remedy or supplement to ensure they are appropriate for individual circumstances and do not interfere with other aspects of diabetes management.

Mind-body techniques for stress management and blood sugar control

Mind-body techniques can be valuable tools for managing stress, promoting relaxation, and potentially helping with blood sugar control in individuals with diabetes. Chronic stress can negatively impact blood sugar levels, so incorporating stress management techniques into a diabetes management plan can be beneficial. Here are some mind-body techniques that may aid in stress reduction and blood sugar control:

1. Meditation: Meditation involves focusing the mind and achieving a state of deep relaxation and mental clarity. Regular meditation practice has been shown to reduce stress, lower blood pressure, and improve overall well-being. It may also have a positive impact on blood sugar control by reducing stress-related hormonal responses.

2. Deep Breathing Exercises: Deep breathing exercises, such as diaphragmatic breathing or "belly breathing," can help activate the body's relaxation response. By taking slow, deep breaths, you can promote a sense of calm and reduce stress. Deep breathing exercises can be practiced anywhere and at any time, making them easily accessible tools for stress management.

3. Yoga: Yoga combines physical postures, breathing exercises, and meditation to promote relaxation, flexibility, and overall mind-body wellness. Regular yoga practice has been associated with reduced stress, improved insulin sensitivity, and better blood sugar control. Certain yoga poses may specifically target the abdominal area, stimulating the pancreas and potentially supporting insulin production.

4. Tai Chi: Tai Chi is an ancient Chinese martial art that involves slow, flowing movements and deep breathing. It promotes relaxation, balance, and mind-body awareness. Tai Chi practice has been linked to reduced stress levels, improved cardiovascular health, and better blood sugar control in individuals with diabetes.

5. Progressive Muscle Relaxation (PMR): PMR involves systematically tensing and relaxing different muscle groups in the body, promoting physical and mental

relaxation. By releasing tension in the muscles, PMR can help reduce stress and improve overall well-being. Regular practice of PMR may contribute to better blood sugar control by managing stress-related hormonal responses.

6. Guided Imagery: Guided imagery involves using visualizations or mental images to evoke a sense of relaxation and calm. It can be practiced through guided audio recordings or with the guidance of a trained professional. Guided imagery can help reduce stress and create a positive mindset, potentially benefiting blood sugar control by minimizing the impact of stress hormones.

Incorporating these mind-body techniques into a daily routine can help individuals with diabetes manage stress, improve their overall well-being, and potentially support blood sugar control. It's important to note that while these techniques may offer benefits, they should not replace standard medical care. It's always advisable to consult with healthcare professionals and diabetes educators to develop a comprehensive diabetes management plan that includes appropriate stress management strategies.

4

Support and Lifestyle Changes

Support and lifestyle changes are crucial for individuals with diabetes to effectively manage their condition and maintain overall health and well-being. Here are some key aspects of support and lifestyle changes that can positively impact diabetes management:

1. Diabetes Education: Diabetes education programs provide individuals with the knowledge and skills necessary to manage their condition effectively. These programs cover topics such as blood sugar monitoring, medication management, healthy eating, physical activity, and problem-solving skills. Diabetes educators and healthcare professionals can guide individuals in understanding their condition and making informed decisions about their lifestyle.

2. Healthcare Team Collaboration: Building a strong relationship with healthcare professionals is vital for ongoing support and guidance. Regular visits to healthcare providers, such as doctors, diabetes educators, dietitians, and endocrinologists, can help individuals track their progress, receive personalized advice, adjust treatment plans, and address any concerns or challenges they may face.

3. Peer Support: Connecting with others who have diabetes can provide a valuable source of support and motivation. Joining diabetes support groups, either in person or online, can create a sense of community, provide opportunities for sharing experiences and tips, and offer emotional support. Peer support can help individuals navigate the challenges of diabetes management and foster a positive mindset.

4. Healthy Eating: Adopting a balanced and nutritious diet is essential for managing

diabetes. A registered dietitian or nutritionist can help develop an individualized meal plan that focuses on portion control, carbohydrate management, fiber-rich foods, and a variety of fruits and vegetables. Choosing whole grains, lean proteins, and healthy fats can help stabilize blood sugar levels, manage weight, and reduce the risk of complications.

5. Regular Physical Activity: Engaging in regular physical activity is beneficial for blood sugar control, weight management, cardiovascular health, and overall well-being. Moderate-intensity activities, such as brisk walking, cycling, swimming, or aerobic exercises, can help improve insulin sensitivity and lower blood sugar levels. It is important to consult with healthcare professionals before starting or modifying an exercise routine, particularly for individuals with pre-existing health conditions.

6. Weight Management: Maintaining a healthy weight is important for individuals with diabetes, as excess body weight can contribute to insulin resistance and blood sugar imbalances. Achieving and maintaining a healthy weight through a combination of balanced eating and regular physical activity can help improve insulin sensitivity and overall glycemic control.

7. Regular Blood Sugar Monitoring: Monitoring blood sugar levels regularly is vital for tracking progress, understanding how lifestyle choices affect blood sugar, and making necessary adjustments to medication, diet, or physical activity. Blood sugar monitoring provides valuable information for individuals and their healthcare team to optimize diabetes management.

8. Stress Management: Chronic stress can impact blood sugar levels, so finding healthy ways to manage stress is important.

Engaging in relaxation techniques, such as meditation, deep breathing exercises, yoga, or engaging in hobbies, can help reduce stress levels and promote overall well-being.

9. Smoking Cessation and Limiting Alcohol Consumption: Smoking and excessive alcohol consumption can have detrimental effects on diabetes management and overall health. Quitting smoking and moderating alcohol intake can help improve blood sugar control, reduce the risk of complications, and enhance overall well-being.

10. Regular Health Check-ups: Regular medical check-ups are essential for monitoring overall health, assessing diabetes-related complications, and adjusting treatment plans as needed. Routine screenings for cholesterol levels, blood pressure, kidney function, eye health, and foot care are important components of comprehensive diabetes management.

By incorporating these support systems and lifestyle changes, individuals with diabetes can effectively manage their condition, improve their quality of life, and reduce the risk of long-term complications. It's important to work closely with healthcare professionals and make personalized adjustments based on individual needs and goals.

The role of healthcare professionals in diabetes reversal

The role of healthcare professionals in diabetes reversal is crucial as they provide guidance, support, and expertise to individuals seeking to reverse or manage their diabetes effectively. Here are some key roles healthcare professionals play in diabetes reversal:

1. Diagnosis and Assessment: Healthcare professionals, such as doctors or endocrinologists, play a vital role in

diagnosing diabetes and determining its severity. They conduct thorough assessments, including blood sugar tests, HbA1c levels, and other relevant diagnostic measures, to understand the individual's current condition and establish a baseline for treatment.

2. Individualized Treatment Plans: Healthcare professionals develop individualized treatment plans based on the specific needs, goals, and medical history of each patient. These plans typically include a combination of medication, lifestyle modifications, and other interventions to help manage or reverse diabetes.

3. Medication Management: Healthcare professionals may prescribe medications to help control blood sugar levels, improve insulin sensitivity, or address specific diabetes-related complications. They monitor the individual's response to medication, adjust dosages as needed, and

educate patients on the proper use, potential side effects, and interactions of the prescribed medications.

4. Nutrition Guidance: Registered dietitians or nutritionists are instrumental in providing dietary guidance to individuals with diabetes. They help develop personalized meal plans that focus on balanced nutrition, portion control, carbohydrate management, and overall healthy eating habits. Healthcare professionals work closely with individuals to educate them about the impact of different foods on blood sugar levels and provide strategies to achieve and maintain a healthy diet.

5. Physical Activity Recommendations: Healthcare professionals, in collaboration with exercise specialists or physiotherapists, provide guidance on the types and intensity of physical activity suitable for individuals with diabetes. They recommend exercise

routines that can help improve insulin sensitivity, promote weight loss or maintenance, and enhance cardiovascular health. These recommendations take into account the individual's fitness level, any existing health conditions, and personal preferences.

6. Continuous Monitoring and Support: Healthcare professionals monitor the progress of individuals undergoing diabetes reversal or management. They regularly assess blood sugar levels, HbA1c values, and other relevant health markers to track improvements and adjust treatment plans accordingly. They provide ongoing support, education, and motivation to individuals, helping them stay on track with their goals and navigate any challenges that arise.

7. Collaboration and Referrals: Healthcare professionals collaborate with other specialists, such as diabetes educators, psychologists, or podiatrists, to provide

comprehensive care. They may refer individuals to specialized healthcare providers as needed to address specific aspects of diabetes management, such as education on self-care techniques, psychological support, or foot care.

8. Education and Self-Management Skills: Healthcare professionals play a crucial role in educating individuals about diabetes, its causes, and the importance of lifestyle modifications for effective management or reversal. They provide guidance on self-monitoring techniques, blood sugar testing, medication management, and problem-solving strategies. They equip individuals with the knowledge and skills necessary to make informed decisions about their health and effectively manage their condition.

Healthcare professionals serve as trusted partners in the journey towards diabetes reversal. Their expertise, ongoing support, and monitoring help individuals achieve better glycemic control, reduce the risk of complications, and improve overall well-being. Regular communication, follow-up appointments, and adherence to recommended treatment plans are key to successful diabetes management and potential reversal.

Building a support system

Building a support system is essential for individuals with diabetes as it provides encouragement, guidance, and understanding throughout their journey. Here are some steps to help build a strong support system:

1. Family and Friends: Start by discussing your diabetes management goals and challenges with your immediate family and close friends. Educate them about the condition and how they can support you. Inform them about signs of high or low

blood sugar levels and how they can assist during emergencies. Encourage them to join you in making healthy lifestyle choices, such as participating in physical activities or preparing nutritious meals together.

2. Diabetes Support Groups: Joining diabetes support groups, either in person or online, can provide a sense of community and understanding. Interacting with others who have similar experiences can offer emotional support, practical advice, and inspiration. These groups may organize meetings, educational sessions, and events that allow you to share experiences, gain knowledge, and build relationships with fellow individuals managing diabetes.

3. Diabetes Educators and Healthcare Providers: Develop a strong relationship with your healthcare team, including diabetes educators, doctors, nurses, dietitians, and pharmacists. They have the expertise to provide guidance, answer

questions, and monitor your progress. Regularly schedule appointments with them to discuss your concerns, receive feedback on your diabetes management, and make any necessary adjustments to your treatment plan.

4. Online Resources and Social Media: Utilize reputable online resources and social media platforms dedicated to diabetes education and support. There are various websites, blogs, forums, and social media groups where you can access valuable information, connect with others managing diabetes, and find inspiration. Ensure that the sources you rely on are credible, evidence-based, and moderated by healthcare professionals or reputable organizations.

5. Diabetes Education Programs: Enroll in diabetes education programs or workshops offered by healthcare facilities, community centers, or organizations focused on

diabetes management. These programs provide valuable information, teach self-management skills, and offer opportunities to connect with others facing similar challenges. You'll learn about blood sugar monitoring, healthy eating, physical activity, medication management, and strategies for coping with diabetes-related issues.

6. Mental Health Support: Don't overlook the importance of mental health in diabetes management. Consider seeking counseling or therapy services to address any emotional challenges or stress related to living with diabetes. Mental health professionals can provide coping strategies, stress management techniques, and help you develop a positive mindset towards managing your condition.

7. Workplace Support: If you feel comfortable, discuss your diabetes management needs with your employer or

human resources department. Inform them about any accommodations you may require, such as flexible work hours for medical appointments or breaks to manage blood sugar levels. This communication can foster understanding and support in your work environment.

Remember, building a support system is an ongoing process. It takes time to find the right individuals and resources that resonate with you. Be open and proactive in seeking support, and don't hesitate to reach out to healthcare professionals or organizations specializing in diabetes care. Having a strong support system can provide the motivation, encouragement, and knowledge necessary to successfully manage diabetes and maintain overall well-being.

Diabetes support groups and communities

Diabetes support groups and communities provide valuable resources, information, and emotional support to individuals living with diabetes. Connecting with others who share similar experiences can be empowering and helpful in managing the challenges of diabetes. Here are some types of diabetes support groups and communities:

1. In-Person Support Groups: In-person support groups bring individuals with diabetes together in a physical location, such as community centers, hospitals, or clinics. These groups often have regular meetings where participants can share their experiences, exchange advice, and provide emotional support. They may also invite guest speakers, such as healthcare professionals or experts in diabetes management, to provide education and guidance.

2. Online Support Communities: Online support communities are forums or social media groups where individuals with

diabetes can connect virtually. These communities allow for 24/7 access to support and information from people worldwide who are managing diabetes. Online platforms provide a space for sharing personal experiences, asking questions, and receiving support from a diverse community of individuals with diabetes.

3. Advocacy Organizations: There are numerous diabetes advocacy organizations that offer support and resources to individuals with diabetes. These organizations often provide online forums, educational materials, webinars, and helplines to address questions and concerns related to diabetes management. They may also organize events, conferences, or local meet-ups to connect individuals with diabetes and provide a platform for advocacy efforts.

4. Diabetes Education Programs: Diabetes education programs, often offered by

healthcare providers or community organizations, provide structured learning and support opportunities. These programs may include group sessions where participants learn about diabetes management techniques, healthy lifestyle choices, and coping strategies. They may also cover topics such as blood sugar monitoring, medication management, and meal planning.

5. Youth and Family Support: Some support groups and communities are specifically tailored to children or adolescents with diabetes and their families. These groups create a safe space for young individuals and their parents to connect, share experiences, and address the unique challenges of managing diabetes in childhood. They often provide education, social activities, and emotional support for both children and parents.

6. Ethnic or Cultural Support Networks: Certain support groups and communities cater to specific ethnic or cultural backgrounds. These groups understand the unique challenges faced by individuals from different cultures and provide support that is culturally sensitive and relevant. They may offer resources in multiple languages, host culturally specific events, and address topics specific to the cultural context of managing diabetes.

7. Peer Mentorship Programs: Peer mentorship programs connect individuals newly diagnosed with diabetes with experienced individuals who can provide guidance, share personal insights, and offer support. This one-on-one connection allows for personalized support and encouragement, helping individuals navigate their diabetes management journey.

It's important to note that while support groups and communities can offer valuable information and emotional support, they should not replace professional medical advice. Always consult with healthcare professionals for personalized guidance and treatment recommendations.

To find diabetes support groups and communities, consider reaching out to local healthcare providers, diabetes clinics, or advocacy organizations. Additionally, online platforms, social media groups, and websites dedicated to diabetes may offer a wealth of resources and connections to virtual support communities.

Coping with the emotional aspects of diabetes

Coping with the emotional aspects of diabetes is an important part of overall diabetes management. Living with a chronic condition like diabetes can bring about various emotional challenges, including stress, frustration, anxiety, and even feelings of sadness or depression. Here are some strategies to help cope with the emotional aspects of diabetes:

1. Education and Understanding: Educate yourself about diabetes to better understand the condition and its management. This knowledge can empower you and reduce uncertainty or fear surrounding the disease. Learn about the factors that influence blood sugar levels, the importance of self-care, and the impact of lifestyle choices. Understanding your condition can help you feel more in control and confident in managing it.

2. Seek Support: Reach out to friends, family, or support groups who can provide understanding and encouragement. Share your experiences, concerns, and triumphs with them. Sometimes just talking about your emotions can provide relief and

perspective. If needed, consider seeking professional help from a therapist or counselor who specializes in chronic illness or diabetes-related mental health.

3. Build a Strong Healthcare Team: Develop a trusting and supportive relationship with your healthcare providers. Regularly communicate with your doctors, nurses, or diabetes educators about your emotional well-being. They can offer guidance, resources, and referrals to mental health professionals if necessary. Collaborate with your healthcare team to create a comprehensive diabetes management plan that addresses both the physical and emotional aspects of your health.

4. Set Realistic Goals: Setting realistic goals and expectations can prevent feelings of overwhelm and frustration. Break down larger goals into smaller, achievable steps. Celebrate your progress along the way, even if it's a small improvement. Recognize that

managing diabetes is a continuous process, and setbacks or fluctuations in blood sugar levels are normal. Be kind to yourself and practice self-compassion.

5. Develop Coping Mechanisms: Identify healthy coping mechanisms to manage stress and emotions. Engage in activities that bring you joy, relaxation, and a sense of calm. This can include hobbies, exercise, meditation, deep breathing exercises, or spending time in nature. Find what works best for you and incorporate it into your daily routine.

6. Connect with Others: Connect with individuals who have diabetes through support groups, online communities, or local events. Sharing experiences with others who understand what you're going through can provide validation, support, and practical tips for coping. Hearing success stories and learning from others can

inspire you and remind you that you are not alone in your journey.

7. Practice Self-Care: Prioritize self-care to nourish your physical, emotional, and mental well-being. This can include getting enough sleep, eating a balanced diet, exercising regularly, and managing stress through relaxation techniques. Engaging in activities that bring you happiness and fulfillment is essential for maintaining a positive mindset and emotional resilience.

8. Monitor Your Mental Health: Pay attention to your mental health and seek help if you notice persistent feelings of sadness, anxiety, or hopelessness. Discuss your emotional well-being with your healthcare team, and don't hesitate to reach out for professional support. Mental health is an integral part of overall well-being, and addressing it can positively impact your diabetes management.

Remember, coping with the emotional aspects of diabetes is an ongoing process. Be patient with yourself and give yourself permission to feel and acknowledge your emotions. With time, self-care, support, and a positive mindset, you can effectively manage the emotional challenges that come with living with diabetes.

Dealing with frustration, fear, and stigma

Dealing with frustration, fear, and stigma related to diabetes can be challenging, but there are strategies to help you navigate these emotions:

1. Educate Yourself and Others: Educate yourself about diabetes and become knowledgeable about the condition. Understanding the facts about diabetes can empower you and help dispel misconceptions. Share accurate information with others, including family, friends, and

colleagues, to combat stigma and promote understanding.

2. Seek Support: Reach out to a support network of individuals who understand and empathize with your experiences. Connect with diabetes support groups, either in-person or online, where you can share your frustrations, fears, and concerns with people who have similar experiences. Being part of a supportive community can provide validation, encouragement, and practical advice.

3. Communicate Openly: Communicate openly with your loved ones, friends, and healthcare providers about your emotions and concerns related to diabetes. Share your frustrations and fears, and express any challenges you may be facing. Open communication can foster understanding, empathy, and support from those around you.

4. Practice Self-Care: Take care of your physical, emotional, and mental well-being. Engage in activities that bring you joy, reduce stress, and promote relaxation. This may include hobbies, exercise, meditation, journaling, or spending time with loved ones. Prioritize self-care to help manage and reduce frustration, fear, and stigma.

5. Challenge Negative Self-Talk: Negative self-talk can worsen feelings of frustration and fear. Be aware of any negative thoughts or self-criticism and challenge them with positive affirmations and realistic perspectives. Remind yourself of your strengths, achievements, and the progress you've made in managing your diabetes.

6. Focus on What You Can Control: Accept that there are factors related to diabetes that are beyond your control. Instead, focus on the aspects you can control, such as adopting a healthy lifestyle, adhering to your treatment plan, and seeking regular

medical care. Taking proactive steps toward self-management can help reduce frustration and fear.

7. Educate Others and Combat Stigma: Take the opportunity to educate others about diabetes whenever possible. Share your personal experiences, correct misconceptions, and advocate for understanding and compassion. By raising awareness and challenging stereotypes, you can help reduce the stigma associated with diabetes.

8. Seek Professional Help: If frustration, fear, or stigma related to diabetes become overwhelming or impact your daily life, consider seeking professional help. A therapist or counselor who specializes in chronic illness or mental health can provide guidance, support, and coping strategies to help you navigate these emotions.

9. Focus on Your Achievements: Celebrate your successes, no matter how small. Recognize the efforts you put into managing your diabetes and the progress you make. Give yourself credit for your resilience and determination. Focusing on your achievements can help counteract feelings of frustration and fear.

10. Advocate for Yourself: Stand up for your rights and needs as a person with diabetes. If you encounter discrimination or stigma in any aspect of your life, be assertive in addressing it. Educate others about your condition and advocate for fair treatment and accommodations when necessary.

Remember, managing frustration, fear, and stigma related to diabetes is an ongoing process. Be patient with yourself and give yourself permission to feel and address these emotions. With support, self-care, and advocacy, you can navigate these challenges and live a fulfilling life while effectively managing your diabetes.

Techniques for improving mental well-being

Improving mental well-being is essential for overall health and can positively impact your ability to manage diabetes. Here are some techniques that can help enhance your mental well-being:

1. Practice Mindfulness and Meditation: Engaging in mindfulness exercises and meditation can help calm your mind, reduce stress, and increase self-awareness. Set aside time each day to focus on the present moment, pay attention to your thoughts and emotions without judgment, and practice deep breathing techniques. Apps and guided meditation resources can be helpful in establishing a regular practice.

2. Engage in Regular Physical Activity: Regular physical activity has numerous mental health benefits. Exercise releases endorphins, which can improve mood and reduce stress. Find physical activities that you enjoy, such as walking, swimming, cycling, dancing, or yoga, and incorporate them into your routine. Aim for at least 150 minutes of moderate-intensity aerobic exercise per week, as recommended by health guidelines.

3. Prioritize Sleep: Good quality sleep is crucial for mental well-being. Establish a consistent sleep routine and create a relaxing environment in your bedroom. Avoid screens and stimulating activities before bedtime, and practice relaxation techniques to help you unwind. If you have trouble sleeping, consult with your healthcare provider for guidance.

4. Build Healthy Relationships: Cultivate meaningful relationships with supportive

and positive people in your life. Surrounding yourself with a strong support system can provide emotional support, reduce feelings of isolation, and contribute to your mental well-being. Foster open communication, spend quality time with loved ones, and seek social connections through support groups or community activities.

5. Practice Self-Care: Take time to care for yourself and engage in activities that bring you joy and relaxation. This can include hobbies, reading, listening to music, taking baths, or practicing self-expression through art or writing. Prioritize self-care as an essential part of your routine and make time for activities that recharge and rejuvenate you.

6. Maintain a Balanced Lifestyle: Strive for a balanced lifestyle that includes healthy eating, regular physical activity, adequate sleep, and stress management. Pay attention to your dietary choices, ensuring they

support your physical and mental well-being. Avoid excessive alcohol consumption and smoking, as they can negatively impact your mental health.

7. Seek Support: Reach out for support when needed. Share your feelings, concerns, and challenges with trusted friends, family members, or a therapist. Professional support can provide guidance, coping strategies, and tools to enhance your mental well-being. Don't hesitate to ask for help when you need it.

8. Challenge Negative Thoughts: Be aware of negative thoughts and challenge them with positive affirmations and realistic perspectives. Practice self-compassion and focus on your strengths and accomplishments. Replace self-criticism with self-encouragement and gratitude for the progress you've made.

9. Limit Stress: Identify sources of stress in your life and develop strategies to manage and reduce them. This may include time management techniques, setting boundaries, practicing relaxation techniques, or seeking stress-reducing activities such as yoga or meditation. Prioritize activities that bring you peace and help you unwind.

10. Seek Professional Help: If you're experiencing persistent feelings of sadness, anxiety, or difficulty coping, consider reaching out to a mental health professional. They can provide specialized support, therapy, and interventions tailored to your specific needs.

Remember that improving mental well-being is an ongoing process. Experiment with different techniques and strategies to find what works best for you. Consistency and self-care are key in maintaining positive mental health and supporting your overall well-being.

5

Long-Term Maintenance and Prevention

Long-term maintenance and prevention are crucial aspects of managing diabetes and reducing the risk of complications. Here are some key strategies for long-term maintenance and prevention:

1. Regular Medical Check-ups: Schedule regular check-ups with your healthcare provider to monitor your diabetes management and overall health. These visits may include blood sugar level monitoring, A1C tests, blood pressure checks, cholesterol level assessments, and foot exams. Regular medical check-ups help detect any potential issues early and allow for timely intervention.

2. Adherence to Medications and Treatment Plans: Follow your healthcare provider's

prescribed treatment plan, including medication regimens, insulin therapy, and lifestyle modifications. Take medications as prescribed, monitor your blood sugar levels regularly, and make any necessary adjustments in consultation with your healthcare team.

3. Healthy Eating Habits: Maintain a well-balanced diet consisting of nutrient-rich foods, including fruits, vegetables, whole grains, lean proteins, and healthy fats. Limit the intake of processed foods, sugary beverages, and foods high in saturated and trans fats. Consider working with a registered dietitian or nutritionist to create a personalized meal plan that aligns with your diabetes management goals.

4. Regular Physical Activity: Engage in regular physical activity to help control blood sugar levels, maintain a healthy weight, and improve overall well-being. Aim for at least 150 minutes of

moderate-intensity aerobic exercise per week, such as brisk walking, cycling, swimming, or dancing. Additionally, incorporate strength training exercises to improve muscle strength and flexibility.

5. Weight Management: Maintain a healthy weight or work towards achieving a healthy weight if necessary. Excess body weight can contribute to insulin resistance and worsen diabetes management. Focus on gradual, sustainable weight loss through a combination of healthy eating, regular physical activity, and behavior modification strategies.

6. Blood Sugar Monitoring: Monitor your blood sugar levels regularly as advised by your healthcare provider. This helps you understand how your body responds to different foods, activities, and medications. Regular monitoring allows for timely adjustments in your diabetes management

plan, helping to maintain stable blood sugar levels.

7. Stress Management: Practice stress management techniques, such as mindfulness, deep breathing exercises, yoga, or engaging in activities that help you relax and unwind. Chronic stress can negatively affect blood sugar control, so finding effective stress management strategies is crucial.

8. Smoking Cessation: If you smoke, quitting is essential for managing diabetes and reducing the risk of complications. Smoking increases the risk of cardiovascular diseases, which can be particularly harmful to individuals with diabetes. Seek support from healthcare professionals, support groups, or smoking cessation programs to help you quit smoking.

9. Regular Eye Exams: Schedule regular eye exams with an eye specialist to monitor for

any diabetes-related eye complications, such as diabetic retinopathy. Early detection and timely intervention can help prevent or slow the progression of vision problems.

10. Foot Care: Take good care of your feet by inspecting them regularly for any cuts, sores, or infections. Keep your feet clean and moisturized, wear comfortable and well-fitting shoes, and avoid going barefoot. Seek prompt medical attention for any foot-related concerns to prevent complications, especially if you have diabetic neuropathy.

11. Diabetes Education and Support: Continue to educate yourself about diabetes management through reputable sources, diabetes education programs, and support groups. Stay updated on the latest research and treatment options. Engage in diabetes self-management education and seek support from healthcare professionals,

diabetes educators, and other individuals living with diabetes.

By incorporating these strategies into your daily routine and actively managing your diabetes, you can reduce the risk of complications, maintain optimal health, and improve your overall quality of life. Remember to consult with your healthcare provider for personalized guidance and to address any specific concerns you may have.

Strategies for maintaining diabetes reversal

Maintaining diabetes reversal involves implementing healthy lifestyle habits and ongoing self-care. Here are some strategies to help you maintain your progress:

1. Healthy Eating Habits: Continue to follow a balanced and nutritious diet that supports your blood sugar control and overall health. Focus on consuming whole, unprocessed

foods, including plenty of fruits, vegetables, whole grains, lean proteins, and healthy fats. Limit the intake of sugary foods, refined carbohydrates, and saturated and trans fats.

2. Portion Control: Practice portion control to ensure you're not overeating. Be mindful of your serving sizes and listen to your body's hunger and fullness cues. Consider using smaller plates, bowls, and utensils to help manage portion sizes effectively.

3. Regular Physical Activity: Maintain an active lifestyle and engage in regular physical activity. Aim for at least 150 minutes of moderate-intensity aerobic exercise per week, along with strength training exercises to maintain muscle mass and bone health. Find activities that you enjoy and make them a part of your routine.

4. Weight Management: Maintain a healthy weight or work towards achieving a healthy

weight if necessary. Weight management is crucial for managing diabetes and reducing the risk of complications. Monitor your weight regularly and make adjustments to your diet and exercise regimen as needed.

5. Blood Sugar Monitoring: Regularly monitor your blood sugar levels as advised by your healthcare provider. This helps you stay aware of any changes and enables you to make necessary adjustments in your diet or medication, if required.

6. Stress Management: Develop effective stress management techniques to minimize the impact of stress on your blood sugar levels. Engage in activities that help you relax, such as meditation, deep breathing exercises, yoga, or hobbies that you enjoy. Prioritize self-care and make time for activities that promote relaxation and well-being.

7. Regular Medical Check-ups: Schedule regular check-ups with your healthcare provider to monitor your health and diabetes management. These visits can help detect any potential issues early and allow for timely intervention or adjustments to your treatment plan.

8. Medication Adherence: If you're on any medications, including those for blood sugar control or other related conditions, ensure you take them as prescribed by your healthcare provider. Follow the recommended dosage and frequency to maintain optimal control of your diabetes.

9. Diabetes Education and Support: Stay educated about diabetes management through reputable sources and continue to seek support from healthcare professionals and diabetes educators. Attend diabetes education programs or support groups to stay informed and connected with others who are managing their diabetes.

10. Lifestyle Modifications: Make healthy lifestyle modifications a permanent part of your routine. Incorporate habits such as regular meal planning, regular physical activity, stress management, and adequate sleep into your daily life. Focus on sustainable changes rather than temporary solutions.

11. Self-Monitoring and Accountability: Stay accountable to yourself by regularly tracking your progress, such as monitoring your weight, blood sugar levels, and physical activity. Keep a journal or use digital tools to record your food intake, exercise, and other relevant information. Self-monitoring can help you stay on track and make necessary adjustments when needed.

12. Celebrate Your Successes: Acknowledge and celebrate your achievements and progress. Recognize the efforts you've put into reversing your diabetes and maintaining a healthy lifestyle. Reward

yourself for reaching milestones and staying committed to your goals.

Remember, maintaining diabetes reversal requires long-term commitment and consistency. It's important to stay motivated, seek support when needed, and make adjustments along the way. Regular communication with your healthcare provider is essential to address any concerns and receive personalized guidance.

Preventing the onset of type 2 diabetes

Preventing the onset of type 2 diabetes involves adopting a healthy lifestyle and making specific behavior changes. Here are some key strategies for preventing type 2 diabetes:

1. Maintain a Healthy Weight: Aim for a healthy weight range by adopting a balanced

diet and engaging in regular physical activity. Losing even a small amount of weight, such as 5-10% of your body weight, can have a significant impact on reducing the risk of developing type 2 diabetes.

2. Follow a Balanced Diet: Emphasize whole, unprocessed foods in your diet, including fruits, vegetables, whole grains, lean proteins, and healthy fats. Limit the intake of sugary foods, refined carbohydrates, processed snacks, and sugary beverages. Focus on portion control and listen to your body's hunger and fullness cues.

3. Be Active: Engage in regular physical activity to help maintain a healthy weight and improve insulin sensitivity. Aim for at least 150 minutes of moderate-intensity aerobic exercise per week, such as brisk walking, cycling, swimming, or dancing. Additionally, incorporate strength training

exercises to build muscle and increase metabolic rate.

4. Make Healthy Beverage Choices: Choose water, herbal tea, or unsweetened beverages instead of sugary drinks like soda, fruit juices, or energy drinks. These sugary beverages can lead to weight gain and increase the risk of developing type 2 diabetes.

5. Manage Stress: Chronic stress can contribute to the development of type 2 diabetes. Find healthy ways to manage stress, such as practicing relaxation techniques, engaging in physical activity, pursuing hobbies, or seeking support from friends, family, or mental health professionals.

6. Get Adequate Sleep: Aim for 7-8 hours of quality sleep each night. Poor sleep habits and insufficient sleep have been linked to an increased risk of developing type 2 diabetes.

Establish a regular sleep routine, create a conducive sleep environment, and prioritize sleep as part of your overall well-being.

7. Quit Smoking: If you smoke, quitting is crucial for reducing the risk of type 2 diabetes, along with other serious health complications. Seek support from healthcare professionals, support groups, or smoking cessation programs to help you quit smoking.

8. Limit Alcohol Intake: If you choose to drink alcohol, do so in moderation. Excessive alcohol consumption can lead to weight gain and increase the risk of developing type 2 diabetes. Follow the recommended guidelines for alcohol consumption, which generally suggest no more than one drink per day for women and two drinks per day for men.

9. Regular Medical Check-ups: Schedule regular check-ups with your healthcare

provider to assess your overall health and monitor any potential risk factors for diabetes. This can include blood sugar level monitoring, blood pressure checks, cholesterol level assessments, and discussions about lifestyle modifications.

10. Diabetes Screening: If you have risk factors for type 2 diabetes, such as a family history of the disease or being overweight, consider undergoing regular diabetes screening tests. Early detection can help identify prediabetes or diabetes at an early stage, allowing for timely intervention and lifestyle modifications.

11. Diabetes Education: Educate yourself about the risk factors, symptoms, and prevention strategies for type 2 diabetes. Attend diabetes education programs or workshops to gain knowledge and practical skills for making healthier choices.

Remember, prevention is key when it comes to type 2 diabetes. By adopting a healthy lifestyle, managing weight, being physically active, and making informed food choices, you can significantly reduce your risk of developing type 2 diabetes. Regular communication with your healthcare provider is essential for personalized guidance and support in your prevention efforts.

Early detection and intervention

Early detection and intervention play a crucial role in managing and preventing complications associated with diabetes. Here are some key aspects of early detection and intervention:

1. Regular Health Check-ups: Schedule regular check-ups with your healthcare provider to monitor your overall health and screen for diabetes risk factors. These check-ups may include measurements of

blood sugar levels, blood pressure, cholesterol levels, and body weight. Early detection of abnormal values can prompt further evaluation and intervention.

2. Diabetes Risk Assessment: Undergo a comprehensive diabetes risk assessment to determine your likelihood of developing diabetes. This assessment may consider factors such as family history, age, weight, physical activity level, and medical history. Identifying your risk level can help guide early intervention strategies.

3. Screening Tests: If you are identified as high-risk based on the diabetes risk assessment, your healthcare provider may recommend specific screening tests. The most common screening test for diabetes is the fasting blood glucose test or the oral glucose tolerance test. These tests help diagnose prediabetes or diabetes at an early stage, allowing for timely intervention.

4. Prediabetes Management: If you are diagnosed with prediabetes, early intervention can help prevent or delay the progression to type 2 diabetes. Prediabetes management typically involves lifestyle modifications, such as adopting a healthy diet, increasing physical activity, and achieving weight loss if necessary. Your healthcare provider may also recommend regular monitoring of blood sugar levels.

5. Medication Intervention: In some cases, medication may be prescribed to manage blood sugar levels in individuals with prediabetes or early-stage diabetes. Medications such as metformin can help improve insulin sensitivity and reduce the risk of progression to diabetes. Your healthcare provider will determine the most appropriate treatment plan based on your individual circumstances.

6. Lifestyle Modifications: Early intervention focuses on adopting healthy

lifestyle habits to manage blood sugar levels and reduce the risk of complications. This includes following a balanced diet, engaging in regular physical activity, managing weight, and implementing stress management techniques. Lifestyle modifications can be effective in controlling blood sugar levels and improving overall health outcomes.

7. Diabetes Education: Receive education and guidance on diabetes self-management from healthcare professionals, diabetes educators, or diabetes support groups. Diabetes education helps individuals understand the condition, learn how to monitor blood sugar levels, manage medications, adopt healthy eating habits, and prevent complications. Education empowers individuals to take an active role in their own health and make informed decisions.

8. Personalized Treatment Plan: Work closely with your healthcare provider to develop a personalized treatment plan based on your individual needs. This plan may involve regular monitoring of blood sugar levels, medication management if necessary, regular check-ups, and ongoing support.

Early detection and intervention are key to managing diabetes effectively and preventing complications. By identifying and addressing diabetes or prediabetes in its early stages, individuals can take proactive steps towards better health outcomes. It's important to maintain regular communication with healthcare professionals, adhere to recommended screenings and tests, and make necessary lifestyle modifications to manage blood sugar levels effectively.

Conclusion

In conclusion, diabetes is a complex chronic condition that requires a comprehensive approach to management and prevention. By implementing key strategies and making important lifestyle changes, individuals can effectively control their blood sugar levels, reduce the risk of complications, and improve their overall health and well-being.

A diabetes-friendly diet, regular physical activity, and weight management are fundamental pillars in diabetes management. Monitoring blood sugar levels and regularly engaging in medical check-ups are vital for early detection and intervention. Medications, including insulin therapy, can be prescribed when necessary to help regulate blood sugar levels. Additionally, alternative therapies, such as herbal remedies and mind-body techniques, may complement conventional treatments.

Building a strong support system, including healthcare professionals, family, and friends, is essential for successful diabetes management. Diabetes support groups and communities can provide valuable resources, information, and emotional support to individuals living with diabetes.

Prevention is also crucial in managing diabetes. Making healthy lifestyle choices, such as adopting a nutritious diet, engaging in regular physical activity, and maintaining a healthy weight, can significantly reduce the risk of developing type 2 diabetes. Early detection through regular screenings and interventions, such as prediabetes management, can help prevent or delay the onset of diabetes.

Coping with the emotional aspects of diabetes, including frustration, fear, and stigma, is an important aspect of overall well-being. Techniques for improving mental well-being, such as stress management and seeking social support, can positively impact both mental and physical health.

In summary, managing diabetes requires a holistic approach that combines medical interventions, lifestyle modifications, and emotional support. By taking proactive steps, individuals with diabetes can lead fulfilling lives, maintain optimal health, and effectively manage their condition. It is crucial to work closely with healthcare professionals and make informed decisions to achieve the best possible outcomes.

Recap of key points

Let's recap the key points discussed in the various aspects of diabetes management and prevention:

1. Diet: Adopt a diabetes-friendly diet that emphasizes balanced meals, portion control, and nutrient-dense foods. Limit the intake

of sugary foods, refined carbohydrates, and processed snacks.

2. Physical Activity: Engage in regular physical activity, including aerobic exercises and strength training, to improve insulin sensitivity and maintain a healthy weight.

3. Blood Sugar Control: Monitor blood glucose levels regularly to track and manage diabetes. This helps in making informed decisions about diet, medication, and lifestyle adjustments.

4. Medications and Insulin Therapy: Depending on individual needs, medications or insulin therapy may be prescribed to manage blood sugar levels effectively.

5. Alternative Therapies: Consider complementary approaches such as herbal remedies, supplements, and mind-body techniques to complement conventional treatments. Consult with healthcare

professionals before incorporating any alternative therapies.

6. Support and Lifestyle Changes: Build a support system consisting of healthcare professionals, family, and friends. Participate in diabetes support groups or communities for valuable resources and emotional support.

7. Prevention: Take steps to prevent the onset of type 2 diabetes by maintaining a healthy weight, following a balanced diet, engaging in physical activity, managing stress, and quitting smoking.

8. Early Detection and Intervention: Undergo regular health check-ups and screenings to detect prediabetes or diabetes at an early stage. Early intervention, including lifestyle modifications and medication if necessary, can help prevent or delay the progression of diabetes.

9. Coping with Emotions: Recognize and address the emotional aspects of living with diabetes by practicing stress management techniques, seeking support, and participating in activities that improve mental well-being.

10. Long-Term Maintenance: Sustain healthy lifestyle habits, continue regular check-ups and screenings, and adhere to recommended treatments to ensure long-term diabetes management and prevention of complications.

Remember, diabetes management is a lifelong journey that requires commitment, education, and support. By incorporating these key points into your daily life, you can effectively manage diabetes, improve your overall health, and reduce the risk of complications. Work closely with healthcare professionals for personalized guidance and support throughout your diabetes journey.

Encouragement and motivation for readers on their journey to reverse type 2 diabetes

To all those embarking on the journey to reverse type 2 diabetes, I want to offer you encouragement and motivation. Reversing diabetes is not an easy task, but it is absolutely possible with dedication and a positive mindset. Remember, you are taking control of your health and making choices that will lead to a better future.

1. Believe in Yourself: You have the power to make a significant change in your life. Believe in your ability to overcome challenges and achieve your goals. Trust that you have the strength and determination to reverse type 2 diabetes.

2. Take it One Step at a Time: Reversing diabetes is a journey that requires patience and persistence. Focus on making small, sustainable changes to your lifestyle.

Celebrate each milestone along the way and remember that progress is not always linear.

3. Stay Positive: Maintaining a positive mindset is crucial throughout your journey. Embrace positivity, even during setbacks. Use any obstacles as learning opportunities and keep pushing forward. Your mindset can greatly influence your success.

4. Find Support: Surround yourself with a strong support system. Seek guidance from healthcare professionals, join diabetes support groups, and lean on family and friends for encouragement. Sharing your journey with others who understand can provide motivation and inspiration.

5. Celebrate Non-Scale Victories: Remember that progress is not just measured by the numbers on the scale or blood sugar readings. Celebrate the non-scale victories, such as having more energy, improved sleep, or fitting into clothes better.

Acknowledge and appreciate the positive changes in your overall well-being.

6. Practice Self-Care: Prioritize self-care and make time for activities that bring you joy and relaxation. Engage in hobbies, practice mindfulness, and take care of your emotional well-being. Self-care supports your overall health and helps you stay focused on your goals.

7. Learn and Educate Yourself: Stay informed about diabetes management and prevention. Educate yourself about nutrition, exercise, and the latest research in diabetes care. Knowledge is power, and being well-informed empowers you to make informed decisions about your health.

8. Celebrate Progress, Not Perfection: Remember that perfection is not the goal. Aim for progress, not perfection. Celebrate even the smallest achievements and keep

building on them. Every positive step you take matters.

9. Visualize Your Success: Envision your life free from the burden of diabetes. Picture yourself achieving your health goals, enjoying an active and vibrant life, and inspiring others with your journey. Visualizing success can help you stay motivated and focused on your ultimate goal.

10. Never Give Up: Lastly, never give up on yourself or your journey to reverse type 2 diabetes. There may be ups and downs, but remember that you are making a life-changing commitment to your health. Stay resilient, keep pushing forward, and trust in your ability to succeed.

You have the power to reverse type 2 diabetes and reclaim your health. Stay committed, stay motivated, and know that you are not alone. Embrace the journey and celebrate every step forward. Your determination and hard work will pay off, and a healthier, diabetes-free future awaits you.

Printed in Great Britain
by Amazon